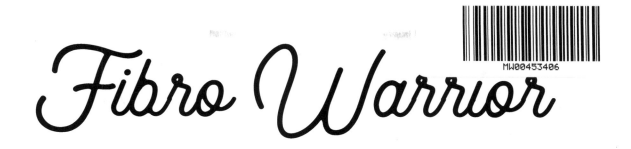

Fibro Warrior

A pain tracking journal

WELLNESS WARRIOR PRESS
www.wellnesswarriorpress.com

Copyright © 2021 by Wellness Warrior Press

ISBN: 978-1-990271-23-6

All rights reserved. No part of this publication may be reproduced, distributed, or transmitted in any form or by any means, including photocopying, recording, or other electronic or mechanical methods, without the prior written permission of the publisher, except in the case of brief quotations embodied in critical reviews and certain other noncommercial uses permitted by copyright law.

This journal belongs to…

_____

DOCTOR / SPECIALIST INFORMATION

Name	Address	Contact

DAILY MEDICATION / SUPPLEMENTS

Medication / Supplement	Dosage

APPOINTMENTS / SURGERIES

Details	Time / Location	Notes

Summary

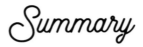

For each journal entry, return to this summary page and rate your overall pain / discomfort level
(1 being no pain and 10 being unbearable)

Entry #	Rating	Entry #	Rating	Entry #	Rating
1		31		61	
2		32		62	
3		33		63	
4		34		64	
5		35		65	
6		36		66	
7		37		67	
8		38		68	
9		39		69	
10		40		70	
11		41		71	
12		42		72	
13		43		73	
14		44		74	
15		45		75	
16		46		76	
17		47		77	
18		48		78	
19		49		79	
20		50		80	
21		51		81	
22		52		82	
23		53		83	
24		54		84	
25		55		85	
26		56		86	
27		57		87	
28		58		88	
29		59		89	
30		60		90	

Summary

For each journal entry, return to this summary page and rate your overall pain / discomfort level
(1 being no pain and 10 being unbearable)

Entry #	Rating	Entry #	Rating	Entry #	Rating
91		121		151	
92		122		152	
93		123		153	
94		124		154	
95		125		155	
96		126		156	
97		127		157	
98		128		158	
99		129		159	
100		130		160	
101		131		161	
102		132		162	
103		133		163	
104		134		164	
105		135		165	
106		136		166	
107		137		167	
108		138		168	
109		139		169	
110		140		170	
111		141		171	
112		142		172	
113		143		173	
114		144		174	
115		145		175	
116		146		176	
117		147		177	
118		148		178	
119		149		179	
120		150		180	

HOW ARE YOU *Feeling today?*

😍 Amazing!	🙂 Meh
😁 Great	😣 Not good
😊 Good	😵 Terrible!

RATE YOUR PAIN LEVEL

① ② ③ ④ ⑤ ⑥ ⑦ ⑧ ⑨ ⑩

WHAT ABOUT YOUR...?

Mood	① ② ③ ④ ⑤ ⑥ ⑦ ⑧ ⑨ ⑩
Energy Levels	① ② ③ ④ ⑤ ⑥ ⑦ ⑧ ⑨ ⑩
Mental Clarity	① ② ③ ④ ⑤ ⑥ ⑦ ⑧ ⑨ ⑩

PAIN & SYMPTOM DETAILS

	am	pm	*front*	*back*	*other*
_____	☐	☐			☐ Nausea
_____	☐	☐			☐ Diarrhea
_____	☐	☐			☐ Vomiting
_____	☐	☐			☐ Sore throat
_____	☐	☐			☐ Congestion
_____	☐	☐			☐ Coughing
_____	☐	☐			☐ Chills
_____	☐	☐			☐ Fever

SLEEP

hours　_____　*quality*　① ② ③ ④ ⑤

STRESS LEVELS

| None | Low | Medium | High | Max | @$#%! |

WEATHER

☐ Cold　☐ Mild　☐ Hot
☐ Dry　☐ Humid　☐ Wet

Allergen Levels: _____
BM Pressure: _____

EXERCISE

☐ Heck yes, I worked out.
☐ I managed to exercise a bit.
☐ No, I haven't exercised at all.
☐ I did some stuff, and that counts.

DETAILS

FOOD / MEDICATION

Food / Drinks

Meds / Supplements	Time	Dose

☐ usual daily medication

Notes
_____
_____

I am grateful for...

HOW ARE YOU *Feeling today?*

😍 Amazing!	🙂 Meh
😁 Great	😠 Not good
🙂 Good	😫 Terrible!

RATE YOUR PAIN LEVEL

① ② ③ ④ ⑤ ⑥ ⑦ ⑧ ⑨ ⑩

WHAT ABOUT YOUR...?

Mood	① ② ③ ④ ⑤ ⑥ ⑦ ⑧ ⑨ ⑩
Energy Levels	① ② ③ ④ ⑤ ⑥ ⑦ ⑧ ⑨ ⑩
Mental Clarity	① ② ③ ④ ⑤ ⑥ ⑦ ⑧ ⑨ ⑩

PAIN & SYMPTOM DETAILS

	am	pm	*front*	*back*	*other*
_____	☐	☐			☐ Nausea
_____	☐	☐			☐ Diarrhea
_____	☐	☐			☐ Vomiting
_____	☐	☐			☐ Sore throat
_____	☐	☐			☐ Congestion
_____	☐	☐			☐ Coughing
_____	☐	☐			☐ Chills
_____	☐	☐			☐ Fever

SLEEP

hours
_____

quality
① ② ③ ④ ⑤

STRESS LEVELS

None	Low	Medium	High	Max	@$#%!

WEATHER

☐ Cold   ☐ Mild   ☐ Hot
☐ Dry   ☐ Humid   ☐ Wet

Allergen Levels: _____
BM Pressure: _____

EXERCISE

☐ Heck yes, I worked out.
☐ I managed to exercise a bit.
☐ No, I haven't exercised at all.
☐ I did some stuff, and that counts.

DETAILS

FOOD / MEDICATION

Food / Drinks

Meds / Supplements	Time	Dose

☐ usual daily medication

Notes
_____
_____

I am grateful for...

HOW ARE YOU *Feeling today?*

😍 Amazing!	🙂 Meh
😁 Great	😣 Not good
😊 Good	😫 Terrible!

RATE YOUR PAIN LEVEL

① ② ③ ④ ⑤ ⑥ ⑦ ⑧ ⑨ ⑩

WHAT ABOUT YOUR...?

Mood	①	②	③	④	⑤	⑥	⑦	⑧	⑨	⑩
Energy Levels	①	②	③	④	⑤	⑥	⑦	⑧	⑨	⑩
Mental Clarity	①	②	③	④	⑤	⑥	⑦	⑧	⑨	⑩

PAIN & SYMPTOM DETAILS

	am	pm	*front*	*back*	*other*
	☐	☐			☐ Nausea
	☐	☐			☐ Diarrhea
	☐	☐			☐ Vomiting
	☐	☐			☐ Sore throat
	☐	☐			☐ Congestion
	☐	☐			☐ Coughing
	☐	☐			☐ Chills
	☐	☐			☐ Fever

SLEEP

hours _____ *quality* ① ② ③ ④ ⑤

STRESS LEVELS

None	Low	Medium	High	Max	@$#%!

WEATHER

☐ Cold ☐ Mild ☐ Hot
☐ Dry ☐ Humid ☐ Wet
Allergen Levels: _____
BM Pressure: _____

EXERCISE

☐ Heck yes, I worked out.
☐ I managed to exercise a bit.
☐ No, I haven't exercised at all.
☐ I did some stuff, and that counts.

DETAILS

FOOD / MEDICATION

Food / Drinks

Meds / Supplements	Time	Dose

☐ usual daily medication

Notes

I am grateful for...

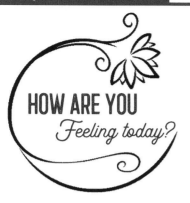

HOW ARE YOU Feeling today?

☺ Amazing!	☺ Meh
☺ Great	☹ Not good
☺ Good	☹ Terrible!

RATE YOUR PAIN LEVEL

① ② ③ ④ ⑤ ⑥ ⑦ ⑧ ⑨ ⑩

WHAT ABOUT YOUR...?

Mood	① ② ③ ④ ⑤ ⑥ ⑦ ⑧ ⑨ ⑩
Energy Levels	① ② ③ ④ ⑤ ⑥ ⑦ ⑧ ⑨ ⑩
Mental Clarity	① ② ③ ④ ⑤ ⑥ ⑦ ⑧ ⑨ ⑩

PAIN & SYMPTOM DETAILS

	am	pm	*front*	*back*	other
	☐	☐			☐ Nausea
	☐	☐			☐ Diarrhea
	☐	☐			☐ Vomiting
	☐	☐			☐ Sore throat
	☐	☐			☐ Congestion
	☐	☐			☐ Coughing
	☐	☐			☐ Chills
	☐	☐			☐ Fever

SLEEP

hours _____

quality ① ② ③ ④ ⑤

STRESS LEVELS

| None | Low | Medium | High | Max | @$#%! |

WEATHER

☐ Cold   ☐ Mild   ☐ Hot
☐ Dry   ☐ Humid   ☐ Wet
Allergen Levels: _____
BM Pressure: _____

EXERCISE

☐ Heck yes, I worked out.
☐ I managed to exercise a bit.
☐ No, I haven't exercised at all.
☐ I did some stuff, and that counts.

DETAILS

FOOD / MEDICATION

Food / Drinks

Meds / Supplements	Time	Dose

☐ usual daily medication

Notes

_____

I am grateful for...

HOW ARE YOU *Feeling today?*

Amazing!	Meh
Great	Not good
Good	Terrible!

RATE YOUR PAIN LEVEL

① ② ③ ④ ⑤ ⑥ ⑦ ⑧ ⑨ ⑩

WHAT ABOUT YOUR...?

Mood	① ② ③ ④ ⑤ ⑥ ⑦ ⑧ ⑨ ⑩
Energy Levels	① ② ③ ④ ⑤ ⑥ ⑦ ⑧ ⑨ ⑩
Mental Clarity	① ② ③ ④ ⑤ ⑥ ⑦ ⑧ ⑨ ⑩

PAIN & SYMPTOM DETAILS

	am	pm	*front*	*back*	*other*
_____	☐	☐			☐ Nausea
_____	☐	☐			☐ Diarrhea
_____	☐	☐			☐ Vomiting
_____	☐	☐			☐ Sore throat
_____	☐	☐			☐ Congestion
_____	☐	☐			☐ Coughing
_____	☐	☐			☐ Chills
_____	☐	☐			☐ Fever

SLEEP

hours   *quality*
_____   ① ② ③ ④ ⑤

STRESS LEVELS

None	Low	Medium	High	Max	@$#%!

WEATHER

☐ Cold   ☐ Mild   ☐ Hot
☐ Dry   ☐ Humid   ☐ Wet
Allergen Levels: _____
BM Pressure: _____

EXERCISE

☐ Heck yes, I worked out.
☐ I managed to exercise a bit.
☐ No, I haven't exercised at all.
☐ I did some stuff, and that counts.

DETAILS

FOOD / MEDICATION

Food / Drinks

Meds / Supplements	Time	Dose

☐ usual daily medication

Notes
_____
_____

I am grateful for...

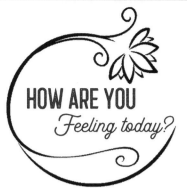

HOW ARE YOU Feeling today?

Amazing!	Meh
Great	Not good
Good	Terrible!

RATE YOUR PAIN LEVEL

① ② ③ ④ ⑤ ⑥ ⑦ ⑧ ⑨ ⑩

WHAT ABOUT YOUR...?

Mood	① ② ③ ④ ⑤ ⑥ ⑦ ⑧ ⑨ ⑩
Energy Levels	① ② ③ ④ ⑤ ⑥ ⑦ ⑧ ⑨ ⑩
Mental Clarity	① ② ③ ④ ⑤ ⑥ ⑦ ⑧ ⑨ ⑩

PAIN & SYMPTOM DETAILS

	am	pm	front	back	other
	☐	☐			☐ Nausea
	☐	☐			☐ Diarrhea
	☐	☐			☐ Vomiting
	☐	☐			☐ Sore throat
	☐	☐			☐ Congestion
	☐	☐			☐ Coughing
	☐	☐			☐ Chills
	☐	☐			☐ Fever

SLEEP

hours
_____

quality
① ② ③ ④ ⑤

STRESS LEVELS

None	Low	Medium	High	Max	@$#%!

WEATHER

☐ Cold ☐ Mild ☐ Hot
☐ Dry ☐ Humid ☐ Wet

Allergen Levels: _____
BM Pressure: _____

EXERCISE

☐ Heck yes, I worked out.
☐ I managed to exercise a bit.
☐ No, I haven't exercised at all.
☐ I did some stuff, and that counts.

DETAILS

FOOD / MEDICATION

Food / Drinks	Meds / Supplements	Time	Dose

☐ usual daily medication

Notes
_____
_____

I am grateful for...

M T W T F S S

DATE:

HOW ARE YOU Feeling today?

😍 Amazing!	🙂 Meh
😁 Great	😠 Not good
😊 Good	😖 Terrible!

RATE YOUR PAIN LEVEL

① ② ③ ④ ⑤ ⑥ ⑦ ⑧ ⑨ ⑩

WHAT ABOUT YOUR...?

Mood	① ② ③ ④ ⑤ ⑥ ⑦ ⑧ ⑨ ⑩
Energy Levels	① ② ③ ④ ⑤ ⑥ ⑦ ⑧ ⑨ ⑩
Mental Clarity	① ② ③ ④ ⑤ ⑥ ⑦ ⑧ ⑨ ⑩

PAIN & SYMPTOM DETAILS

	am	pm	front	back	other
	☐	☐			☐ Nausea
	☐	☐			☐ Diarrhea
	☐	☐			☐ Vomiting
	☐	☐			☐ Sore throat
	☐	☐			☐ Congestion
	☐	☐			☐ Coughing
	☐	☐			☐ Chills
	☐	☐			☐ Fever

SLEEP

hours
_____

quality
① ② ③ ④ ⑤

STRESS LEVELS

None	Low	Medium	High	Max	@$#%!

WEATHER

☐ Cold   ☐ Mild   ☐ Hot
☐ Dry   ☐ Humid   ☐ Wet

Allergen Levels: _____
BM Pressure: _____

EXERCISE

☐ Heck yes, I worked out.
☐ I managed to exercise a bit.
☐ No, I haven't exercised at all.
☐ I did some stuff, and that counts.

DETAILS

FOOD / MEDICATION

Food / Drinks

Meds / Supplements	Time	Dose

☐ usual daily medication

Notes
_____

I am grateful for...
_____

M T W T F S S DATE:

HOW ARE YOU *Feeling today?*

Amazing!	Meh
Great	Not good
Good	Terrible!

RATE YOUR PAIN LEVEL

① ② ③ ④ ⑤ ⑥ ⑦ ⑧ ⑨ ⑩

WHAT ABOUT YOUR...?

Mood	① ② ③ ④ ⑤ ⑥ ⑦ ⑧ ⑨ ⑩
Energy Levels	① ② ③ ④ ⑤ ⑥ ⑦ ⑧ ⑨ ⑩
Mental Clarity	① ② ③ ④ ⑤ ⑥ ⑦ ⑧ ⑨ ⑩

PAIN & SYMPTOM DETAILS

	am	pm	front	back	other
	☐	☐			☐ Nausea
	☐	☐			☐ Diarrhea
	☐	☐			☐ Vomiting
	☐	☐			☐ Sore throat
	☐	☐			☐ Congestion
	☐	☐			☐ Coughing
	☐	☐			☐ Chills
	☐	☐			☐ Fever

SLEEP

hours
_____

quality
① ② ③ ④ ⑤

STRESS LEVELS

None	Low	Medium	High	Max	@$#%!

WEATHER

☐ Cold   ☐ Mild   ☐ Hot
☐ Dry   ☐ Humid ☐ Wet

Allergen Levels: _____
BM Pressure: _____

EXERCISE

☐ Heck yes, I worked out.
☐ I managed to exercise a bit.
☐ No, I haven't exercised at all.
☐ I did some stuff, and that counts.

DETAILS

FOOD / MEDICATION

Food / Drinks

Meds / Supplements	Time	Dose

☐ usual daily medication

Notes
_____

I am grateful for...
_____

M T W T F S S   DATE:

HOW ARE YOU Feeling today?

Amazing!	Meh
Great	Not good
Good	Terrible!

RATE YOUR PAIN LEVEL

① ② ③ ④ ⑤ ⑥ ⑦ ⑧ ⑨ ⑩

WHAT ABOUT YOUR...?

Mood	①	②	③	④	⑤	⑥	⑦	⑧	⑨	⑩
Energy Levels	①	②	③	④	⑤	⑥	⑦	⑧	⑨	⑩
Mental Clarity	①	②	③	④	⑤	⑥	⑦	⑧	⑨	⑩

PAIN & SYMPTOM DETAILS

	am	pm	front	back	other
_____	☐	☐			☐ Nausea
_____	☐	☐			☐ Diarrhea
_____	☐	☐			☐ Vomiting
_____	☐	☐			☐ Sore throat
_____	☐	☐			☐ Congestion
_____	☐	☐			☐ Coughing
_____	☐	☐			☐ Chills
_____	☐	☐			☐ Fever

SLEEP

hours
_____

quality
① ② ③ ④ ⑤

STRESS LEVELS

None	Low	Medium	High	Max	@$#%!

WEATHER

☐ Cold   ☐ Mild   ☐ Hot
☐ Dry   ☐ Humid   ☐ Wet
Allergen Levels: _____
BM Pressure: _____

EXERCISE

☐ Heck yes, I worked out.
☐ I managed to exercise a bit.
☐ No, I haven't exercised at all.
☐ I did some stuff, and that counts.

DETAILS

FOOD / MEDICATION

Food / Drinks	Meds / Supplements	Time	Dose

☐ usual daily medication

Notes
_____
_____

I am grateful for...

HOW ARE YOU *Feeling today?*

😍 Amazing!	🙂 Meh
😁 Great	😠 Not good
🙂 Good	😣 Terrible!

RATE YOUR PAIN LEVEL

① ② ③ ④ ⑤ ⑥ ⑦ ⑧ ⑨ ⑩

WHAT ABOUT YOUR...?

Mood	① ② ③ ④ ⑤ ⑥ ⑦ ⑧ ⑨ ⑩
Energy Levels	① ② ③ ④ ⑤ ⑥ ⑦ ⑧ ⑨ ⑩
Mental Clarity	① ② ③ ④ ⑤ ⑥ ⑦ ⑧ ⑨ ⑩

PAIN & SYMPTOM DETAILS

	am	pm	*front*	*back*	other
_____	☐	☐			☐ Nausea
_____	☐	☐			☐ Diarrhea
_____	☐	☐			☐ Vomiting
_____	☐	☐			☐ Sore throat
_____	☐	☐			☐ Congestion
_____	☐	☐			☐ Coughing
_____	☐	☐			☐ Chills
_____	☐	☐			☐ Fever

SLEEP

hours
_____

quality
① ② ③ ④ ⑤

STRESS LEVELS

None	Low	Medium	High	Max	@$#%!

WEATHER

☐ Cold   ☐ Mild   ☐ Hot
☐ Dry   ☐ Humid ☐ Wet
Allergen Levels: _____
BM Pressure: _____

EXERCISE

☐ Heck yes, I worked out.
☐ I managed to exercise a bit.
☐ No, I haven't exercised at all.
☐ I did some stuff, and that counts.

DETAILS

FOOD / MEDICATION

Food / Drinks

Meds / Supplements	Time	Dose

☐ usual daily medication

Notes
_____
_____

I am grateful for...

M T W T F S S

DATE:

HOW ARE YOU Feeling today?

😍 Amazing!	🙂 Meh
😁 Great	😣 Not good
😊 Good	😫 Terrible!

RATE YOUR PAIN LEVEL

① ② ③ ④ ⑤ ⑥ ⑦ ⑧ ⑨ ⑩

WHAT ABOUT YOUR...?

Mood	① ② ③ ④ ⑤ ⑥ ⑦ ⑧ ⑨ ⑩
Energy Levels	① ② ③ ④ ⑤ ⑥ ⑦ ⑧ ⑨ ⑩
Mental Clarity	① ② ③ ④ ⑤ ⑥ ⑦ ⑧ ⑨ ⑩

PAIN & SYMPTOM DETAILS

	am	pm	front	back	other
	☐	☐			☐ Nausea
	☐	☐			☐ Diarrhea
	☐	☐			☐ Vomiting
	☐	☐			☐ Sore throat
	☐	☐			☐ Congestion
	☐	☐			☐ Coughing
	☐	☐			☐ Chills
	☐	☐			☐ Fever

SLEEP

hours _____

quality ① ② ③ ④ ⑤

STRESS LEVELS

None	Low	Medium	High	Max	@$#%!

WEATHER

☐ Cold   ☐ Mild   ☐ Hot
☐ Dry   ☐ Humid   ☐ Wet
Allergen Levels: _____
BM Pressure: _____

EXERCISE

☐ Heck yes, I worked out.
☐ I managed to exercise a bit.
☐ No, I haven't exercised at all.
☐ I did some stuff, and that counts.

DETAILS

FOOD / MEDICATION

Food / Drinks

Meds / Supplements	Time	Dose

☐ usual daily medication

Notes

I am grateful for…

HOW ARE YOU *Feeling today?*

😍 Amazing!	🙂 Meh
😁 Great	😠 Not good
🙂 Good	😫 Terrible!

RATE YOUR PAIN LEVEL

① ② ③ ④ ⑤ ⑥ ⑦ ⑧ ⑨ ⑩

WHAT ABOUT YOUR...?

Mood	① ② ③ ④ ⑤ ⑥ ⑦ ⑧ ⑨ ⑩
Energy Levels	① ② ③ ④ ⑤ ⑥ ⑦ ⑧ ⑨ ⑩
Mental Clarity	① ② ③ ④ ⑤ ⑥ ⑦ ⑧ ⑨ ⑩

PAIN & SYMPTOM DETAILS

	am	pm	front	back	other
_____	☐	☐			☐ Nausea
_____	☐	☐			☐ Diarrhea
_____	☐	☐			☐ Vomiting
_____	☐	☐			☐ Sore throat
_____	☐	☐			☐ Congestion
_____	☐	☐			☐ Coughing
_____	☐	☐			☐ Chills
_____	☐	☐			☐ Fever

SLEEP

hours
_____

quality
① ② ③ ④ ⑤

STRESS LEVELS

None	Low	Medium	High	Max	@$#%!

WEATHER

☐ Cold   ☐ Mild   ☐ Hot
☐ Dry   ☐ Humid   ☐ Wet

Allergen Levels: _____
BM Pressure: _____

EXERCISE

☐ Heck yes, I worked out.
☐ I managed to exercise a bit.
☐ No, I haven't exercised at all.
☐ I did some stuff, and that counts.

DETAILS

FOOD / MEDICATION

Food / Drinks

Meds / Supplements	Time	Dose

☐ usual daily medication

Notes
_____

_____

I am grateful for...

M T W T F S S   DATE:

HOW ARE YOU *Feeling today?*

😍 Amazing!	🙂 Meh
😁 Great	😣 Not good
😊 Good	😫 Terrible!

RATE YOUR PAIN LEVEL

① ② ③ ④ ⑤ ⑥ ⑦ ⑧ ⑨ ⑩

WHAT ABOUT YOUR...?

Mood	① ② ③ ④ ⑤ ⑥ ⑦ ⑧ ⑨ ⑩
Energy Levels	① ② ③ ④ ⑤ ⑥ ⑦ ⑧ ⑨ ⑩
Mental Clarity	① ② ③ ④ ⑤ ⑥ ⑦ ⑧ ⑨ ⑩

PAIN & SYMPTOM DETAILS

	am	pm	front	back	other
_____	☐	☐			☐ Nausea
_____	☐	☐			☐ Diarrhea
_____	☐	☐			☐ Vomiting
_____	☐	☐			☐ Sore throat
_____	☐	☐			☐ Congestion
_____	☐	☐			☐ Coughing
_____	☐	☐			☐ Chills
_____	☐	☐			☐ Fever

SLEEP

hours
_____

quality
① ② ③ ④ ⑤

STRESS LEVELS

None	Low	Medium	High	Max	@$#%!

WEATHER

☐ Cold ☐ Mild ☐ Hot
☐ Dry ☐ Humid ☐ Wet
Allergen Levels: _____
BM Pressure: _____

EXERCISE

☐ Heck yes, I worked out.
☐ I managed to exercise a bit.
☐ No, I haven't exercised at all.
☐ I did some stuff, and that counts.

DETAILS

FOOD / MEDICATION

Food / Drinks

Meds / Supplements	Time	Dose

☐ usual daily medication

Notes
_____
_____

I am grateful for...

M T W T F S S   DATE:

HOW ARE YOU *Feeling today?*

Amazing!	Meh
Great	Not good
Good	Terrible!

RATE YOUR PAIN LEVEL

① ② ③ ④ ⑤ ⑥ ⑦ ⑧ ⑨ ⑩

WHAT ABOUT YOUR...?

Mood	① ② ③ ④ ⑤ ⑥ ⑦ ⑧ ⑨ ⑩
Energy Levels	① ② ③ ④ ⑤ ⑥ ⑦ ⑧ ⑨ ⑩
Mental Clarity	① ② ③ ④ ⑤ ⑥ ⑦ ⑧ ⑨ ⑩

PAIN & SYMPTOM DETAILS

	am	pm	*front*	*back*	*other*
_____	☐	☐			☐ Nausea
_____	☐	☐			☐ Diarrhea
_____	☐	☐			☐ Vomiting
_____	☐	☐			☐ Sore throat
_____	☐	☐			☐ Congestion
_____	☐	☐			☐ Coughing
_____	☐	☐			☐ Chills
_____	☐	☐			☐ Fever

SLEEP

hours
_____

quality
① ② ③ ④ ⑤

STRESS LEVELS

None	Low	Medium	High	Max	@$#%!

WEATHER

☐ Cold   ☐ Mild   ☐ Hot
☐ Dry   ☐ Humid   ☐ Wet
Allergen Levels: _____
BM Pressure: _____

EXERCISE

☐ Heck yes, I worked out.
☐ I managed to exercise a bit.
☐ No, I haven't exercised at all.
☐ I did some stuff, and that counts.

DETAILS

FOOD / MEDICATION

Food / Drinks

Meds / Supplements	Time	Dose

☐ usual daily medication

Notes
_____
_____

I am grateful for...

HOW ARE YOU *Feeling today?*

😍 Amazing!	🙂 Meh
😁 Great	😠 Not good
😊 Good	😖 Terrible!

RATE YOUR PAIN LEVEL

① ② ③ ④ ⑤ ⑥ ⑦ ⑧ ⑨ ⑩

WHAT ABOUT YOUR...?

Mood	① ② ③ ④ ⑤ ⑥ ⑦ ⑧ ⑨ ⑩
Energy Levels	① ② ③ ④ ⑤ ⑥ ⑦ ⑧ ⑨ ⑩
Mental Clarity	① ② ③ ④ ⑤ ⑥ ⑦ ⑧ ⑨ ⑩

PAIN & SYMPTOM DETAILS

	am	pm	front	back	other
	☐	☐			☐ Nausea
	☐	☐			☐ Diarrhea
	☐	☐			☐ Vomiting
	☐	☐			☐ Sore throat
	☐	☐			☐ Congestion
	☐	☐			☐ Coughing
	☐	☐			☐ Chills
	☐	☐			☐ Fever

SLEEP

hours _____ *quality* ① ② ③ ④ ⑤

STRESS LEVELS

None	Low	Medium	High	Max	@$#%!

WEATHER

☐ Cold   ☐ Mild   ☐ Hot
☐ Dry   ☐ Humid   ☐ Wet
Allergen Levels: _____
BM Pressure: _____

EXERCISE

☐ Heck yes, I worked out.
☐ I managed to exercise a bit.
☐ No, I haven't exercised at all.
☐ I did some stuff, and that counts.

DETAILS

FOOD / MEDICATION

Food / Drinks

Meds / Supplements	Time	Dose

☐ usual daily medication

Notes

I am grateful for...

M T W T F S S   DATE:

HOW ARE YOU Feeling today?

Amazing!	Meh
Great	Not good
Good	Terrible!

RATE YOUR PAIN LEVEL

1 2 3 4 5 6 7 8 9 10

WHAT ABOUT YOUR...?

Mood	1 2 3 4 5 6 7 8 9 10
Energy Levels	1 2 3 4 5 6 7 8 9 10
Mental Clarity	1 2 3 4 5 6 7 8 9 10

PAIN & SYMPTOM DETAILS

	am	pm	front	back	other
	☐	☐			☐ Nausea
	☐	☐			☐ Diarrhea
	☐	☐			☐ Vomiting
	☐	☐			☐ Sore throat
	☐	☐			☐ Congestion
	☐	☐			☐ Coughing
	☐	☐			☐ Chills
	☐	☐			☐ Fever

SLEEP

hours   *quality*
_____   1 2 3 4 5

STRESS LEVELS

None	Low	Medium	High	Max	@$#%!

WEATHER

☐ Cold   ☐ Mild   ☐ Hot
☐ Dry   ☐ Humid   ☐ Wet
Allergen Levels: _____
BM Pressure: _____

EXERCISE

☐ Heck yes, I worked out.
☐ I managed to exercise a bit.
☐ No, I haven't exercised at all.
☐ I did some stuff, and that counts.

DETAILS

FOOD / MEDICATION

Food / Drinks

Meds / Supplements	Time	Dose

☐ usual daily medication

Notes

I am grateful for...

HOW ARE YOU *Feeling today?*

😍 Amazing!	🙂 Meh
😁 Great	😣 Not good
😊 Good	😖 Terrible!

RATE YOUR PAIN LEVEL

① ② ③ ④ ⑤ ⑥ ⑦ ⑧ ⑨ ⑩

WHAT ABOUT YOUR...?

Mood	① ② ③ ④ ⑤ ⑥ ⑦ ⑧ ⑨ ⑩
Energy Levels	① ② ③ ④ ⑤ ⑥ ⑦ ⑧ ⑨ ⑩
Mental Clarity	① ② ③ ④ ⑤ ⑥ ⑦ ⑧ ⑨ ⑩

PAIN & SYMPTOM DETAILS

	am	pm	*front*	*back*	*other*
_____	☐	☐			☐ Nausea
_____	☐	☐			☐ Diarrhea
_____	☐	☐			☐ Vomiting
_____	☐	☐			☐ Sore throat
_____	☐	☐			☐ Congestion
_____	☐	☐			☐ Coughing
_____	☐	☐			☐ Chills
_____	☐	☐			☐ Fever

SLEEP

hours _____

quality ① ② ③ ④ ⑤

STRESS LEVELS

None	Low	Medium	High	Max	@$#%!

WEATHER

☐ Cold   ☐ Mild   ☐ Hot
☐ Dry   ☐ Humid   ☐ Wet
Allergen Levels: _____
BM Pressure: _____

EXERCISE

☐ Heck yes, I worked out.
☐ I managed to exercise a bit.
☐ No, I haven't exercised at all.
☐ I did some stuff, and that counts.

DETAILS

FOOD / MEDICATION

Food / Drinks

Meds / Supplements	Time	Dose

☐ usual daily medication

Notes
_____
_____

I am grateful for...

HOW ARE YOU *Feeling today?*

Amazing!	Meh
Great	Not good
Good	Terrible!

RATE YOUR PAIN LEVEL

① ② ③ ④ ⑤ ⑥ ⑦ ⑧ ⑨ ⑩

WHAT ABOUT YOUR...?

Mood	① ② ③ ④ ⑤ ⑥ ⑦ ⑧ ⑨ ⑩
Energy Levels	① ② ③ ④ ⑤ ⑥ ⑦ ⑧ ⑨ ⑩
Mental Clarity	① ② ③ ④ ⑤ ⑥ ⑦ ⑧ ⑨ ⑩

PAIN & SYMPTOM DETAILS

	am	pm	*front*	*back*	*other*
	☐	☐			☐ Nausea
	☐	☐			☐ Diarrhea
	☐	☐			☐ Vomiting
	☐	☐			☐ Sore throat
	☐	☐			☐ Congestion
	☐	☐			☐ Coughing
	☐	☐			☐ Chills
	☐	☐			☐ Fever

SLEEP

hours _____

quality ① ② ③ ④ ⑤

STRESS LEVELS

None	Low	Medium	High	Max	@$#%!

WEATHER

☐ Cold   ☐ Mild   ☐ Hot
☐ Dry   ☐ Humid   ☐ Wet

Allergen Levels: _____
BM Pressure: _____

EXERCISE

☐ Heck yes, I worked out.
☐ I managed to exercise a bit.
☐ No, I haven't exercised at all.
☐ I did some stuff, and that counts.

DETAILS

FOOD / MEDICATION

Food / Drinks	Meds / Supplements	Time	Dose

☐ usual daily medication

Notes

I am grateful for...

HOW ARE YOU *Feeling today?*

😍 Amazing!	🙂 Meh
😁 Great	😠 Not good
😊 Good	😖 Terrible!

RATE YOUR PAIN LEVEL

① ② ③ ④ ⑤ ⑥ ⑦ ⑧ ⑨ ⑩

WHAT ABOUT YOUR...?

Mood	①	②	③	④	⑤	⑥	⑦	⑧	⑨	⑩
Energy Levels	①	②	③	④	⑤	⑥	⑦	⑧	⑨	⑩
Mental Clarity	①	②	③	④	⑤	⑥	⑦	⑧	⑨	⑩

PAIN & SYMPTOM DETAILS

	am	pm	front	back	other
_____	☐	☐			☐ Nausea
_____	☐	☐			☐ Diarrhea
_____	☐	☐			☐ Vomiting
_____	☐	☐			☐ Sore throat
_____	☐	☐			☐ Congestion
_____	☐	☐			☐ Coughing
_____	☐	☐			☐ Chills
_____	☐	☐			☐ Fever

SLEEP

hours _____

quality ① ② ③ ④ ⑤

STRESS LEVELS

None	Low	Medium	High	Max	@$#%!

WEATHER

☐ Cold   ☐ Mild   ☐ Hot
☐ Dry   ☐ Humid   ☐ Wet

Allergen Levels: _____
BM Pressure: _____

EXERCISE

☐ Heck yes, I worked out.
☐ I managed to exercise a bit.
☐ No, I haven't exercised at all.
☐ I did some stuff, and that counts.

DETAILS

FOOD / MEDICATION

Food / Drinks

Meds / Supplements	Time	Dose

☐ usual daily medication

Notes
_____

I am grateful for...

HOW ARE YOU Feeling today?

Amazing!	Meh
Great	Not good
Good	Terrible!

RATE YOUR PAIN LEVEL

① ② ③ ④ ⑤ ⑥ ⑦ ⑧ ⑨ ⑩

WHAT ABOUT YOUR...?

Mood	① ② ③ ④ ⑤ ⑥ ⑦ ⑧ ⑨ ⑩
Energy Levels	① ② ③ ④ ⑤ ⑥ ⑦ ⑧ ⑨ ⑩
Mental Clarity	① ② ③ ④ ⑤ ⑥ ⑦ ⑧ ⑨ ⑩

PAIN & SYMPTOM DETAILS

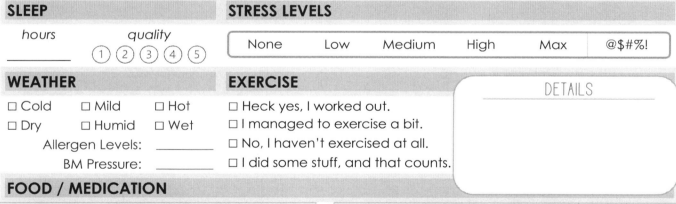

	am	pm		*front*	*back*		other
	☐	☐					☐ Nausea
	☐	☐					☐ Diarrhea
	☐	☐					☐ Vomiting
	☐	☐					☐ Sore throat
	☐	☐					☐ Congestion
	☐	☐					☐ Coughing
	☐	☐					☐ Chills
	☐	☐					☐ Fever

SLEEP

hours _____   *quality* ① ② ③ ④ ⑤

STRESS LEVELS

None	Low	Medium	High	Max	@$#%!

WEATHER

☐ Cold   ☐ Mild   ☐ Hot
☐ Dry   ☐ Humid   ☐ Wet
Allergen Levels: _____
BM Pressure: _____

EXERCISE

☐ Heck yes, I worked out.
☐ I managed to exercise a bit.
☐ No, I haven't exercised at all.
☐ I did some stuff, and that counts.

DETAILS

FOOD / MEDICATION

Food / Drinks

Meds / Supplements	Time	Dose

☐ usual daily medication

Notes

I am grateful for...

HOW ARE YOU Feeling today?

Amazing!	Meh
Great	Not good
Good	Terrible!

RATE YOUR PAIN LEVEL

① ② ③ ④ ⑤ ⑥ ⑦ ⑧ ⑨ ⑩

WHAT ABOUT YOUR...?

Mood	① ② ③ ④ ⑤ ⑥ ⑦ ⑧ ⑨ ⑩
Energy Levels	① ② ③ ④ ⑤ ⑥ ⑦ ⑧ ⑨ ⑩
Mental Clarity	① ② ③ ④ ⑤ ⑥ ⑦ ⑧ ⑨ ⑩

PAIN & SYMPTOM DETAILS

	am	pm	front	back	other
	☐	☐			☐ Nausea
	☐	☐			☐ Diarrhea
	☐	☐			☐ Vomiting
	☐	☐			☐ Sore throat
	☐	☐			☐ Congestion
	☐	☐			☐ Coughing
	☐	☐			☐ Chills
	☐	☐			☐ Fever

SLEEP

hours _____

quality ① ② ③ ④ ⑤

STRESS LEVELS

None	Low	Medium	High	Max	@$#%!

WEATHER

☐ Cold ☐ Mild ☐ Hot
☐ Dry   ☐ Humid ☐ Wet
Allergen Levels: _____
BM Pressure: _____

EXERCISE

☐ Heck yes, I worked out.
☐ I managed to exercise a bit.
☐ No, I haven't exercised at all.
☐ I did some stuff, and that counts.

DETAILS

FOOD / MEDICATION

Food / Drinks

Meds / Supplements	Time	Dose

☐ usual daily medication

Notes
_____
_____

I am grateful for…

HOW ARE YOU *Feeling today?*

😍 Amazing!	🙂 Meh
😁 Great	😠 Not good
🙂 Good	😖 Terrible!

RATE YOUR PAIN LEVEL

① ② ③ ④ ⑤ ⑥ ⑦ ⑧ ⑨ ⑩

WHAT ABOUT YOUR...?

Mood	① ② ③ ④ ⑤ ⑥ ⑦ ⑧ ⑨ ⑩
Energy Levels	① ② ③ ④ ⑤ ⑥ ⑦ ⑧ ⑨ ⑩
Mental Clarity	① ② ③ ④ ⑤ ⑥ ⑦ ⑧ ⑨ ⑩

PAIN & SYMPTOM DETAILS

	am	pm	*front*	*back*	*other*
_____	☐	☐			☐ Nausea
_____	☐	☐			☐ Diarrhea
_____	☐	☐			☐ Vomiting
_____	☐	☐			☐ Sore throat
_____	☐	☐			☐ Congestion
_____	☐	☐			☐ Coughing
_____	☐	☐			☐ Chills
_____	☐	☐			☐ Fever

SLEEP

hours
_____

quality
① ② ③ ④ ⑤

STRESS LEVELS

None	Low	Medium	High	Max	@$#%!

WEATHER

☐ Cold   ☐ Mild   ☐ Hot
☐ Dry   ☐ Humid   ☐ Wet

Allergen Levels: _____
BM Pressure: _____

EXERCISE

☐ Heck yes, I worked out.
☐ I managed to exercise a bit.
☐ No, I haven't exercised at all.
☐ I did some stuff, and that counts.

DETAILS

FOOD / MEDICATION

Food / Drinks

Meds / Supplements	Time	Dose

☐ usual daily medication

Notes

I am grateful for...

HOW ARE YOU Feeling today?

😍 Amazing!	🙂 Meh
😁 Great	😠 Not good
😊 Good	😖 Terrible!

RATE YOUR PAIN LEVEL

① ② ③ ④ ⑤ ⑥ ⑦ ⑧ ⑨ ⑩

WHAT ABOUT YOUR...?

Mood	① ② ③ ④ ⑤ ⑥ ⑦ ⑧ ⑨ ⑩
Energy Levels	① ② ③ ④ ⑤ ⑥ ⑦ ⑧ ⑨ ⑩
Mental Clarity	① ② ③ ④ ⑤ ⑥ ⑦ ⑧ ⑨ ⑩

PAIN & SYMPTOM DETAILS

	am	pm	front	back	other
_____	☐	☐			☐ Nausea
_____	☐	☐			☐ Diarrhea
_____	☐	☐			☐ Vomiting
_____	☐	☐			☐ Sore throat
_____	☐	☐			☐ Congestion
_____	☐	☐			☐ Coughing
_____	☐	☐			☐ Chills
_____	☐	☐			☐ Fever

SLEEP

hours
_____

quality
① ② ③ ④ ⑤

STRESS LEVELS

None	Low	Medium	High	Max	@$#%!

WEATHER

☐ Cold   ☐ Mild   ☐ Hot
☐ Dry   ☐ Humid ☐ Wet
Allergen Levels: _____
BM Pressure: _____

EXERCISE

☐ Heck yes, I worked out.
☐ I managed to exercise a bit.
☐ No, I haven't exercised at all.
☐ I did some stuff, and that counts.

DETAILS

FOOD / MEDICATION

Food / Drinks

Meds / Supplements	Time	Dose

☐ usual daily medication

Notes
_____
_____

I am grateful for...

HOW ARE YOU *Feeling today?*

😍 Amazing!	🙂 Meh
😁 Great	😠 Not good
🙂 Good	😣 Terrible!

RATE YOUR PAIN LEVEL

① ② ③ ④ ⑤ ⑥ ⑦ ⑧ ⑨ ⑩

WHAT ABOUT YOUR...?

Mood	① ② ③ ④ ⑤ ⑥ ⑦ ⑧ ⑨ ⑩
Energy Levels	① ② ③ ④ ⑤ ⑥ ⑦ ⑧ ⑨ ⑩
Mental Clarity	① ② ③ ④ ⑤ ⑥ ⑦ ⑧ ⑨ ⑩

PAIN & SYMPTOM DETAILS

	am	pm	*front*	*back*	*other*
_____	☐	☐			☐ Nausea
_____	☐	☐			☐ Diarrhea
_____	☐	☐			☐ Vomiting
_____	☐	☐			☐ Sore throat
_____	☐	☐			☐ Congestion
_____	☐	☐			☐ Coughing
_____	☐	☐			☐ Chills
_____	☐	☐			☐ Fever

SLEEP

hours
_____

quality
① ② ③ ④ ⑤

STRESS LEVELS

None	Low	Medium	High	Max	@$#%!

WEATHER

☐ Cold   ☐ Mild   ☐ Hot
☐ Dry   ☐ Humid   ☐ Wet
Allergen Levels: _____
BM Pressure: _____

EXERCISE

☐ Heck yes, I worked out.
☐ I managed to exercise a bit.
☐ No, I haven't exercised at all.
☐ I did some stuff, and that counts.

DETAILS

FOOD / MEDICATION

Food / Drinks

Meds / Supplements	Time	Dose

☐ usual daily medication

Notes
_____
_____

I am grateful for...

M T W T F S S   DATE:

HOW ARE YOU
Feeling today?

😍 Amazing!	🙂 Meh
😁 Great	😣 Not good
😊 Good	😵 Terrible!

RATE YOUR PAIN LEVEL

(1) (2) (3) (4) (5) (6) (7) (8) (9) (10)

WHAT ABOUT YOUR...?

Mood	(1) (2) (3) (4) (5) (6) (7) (8) (9) (10)
Energy Levels	(1) (2) (3) (4) (5) (6) (7) (8) (9) (10)
Mental Clarity	(1) (2) (3) (4) (5) (6) (7) (8) (9) (10)

PAIN & SYMPTOM DETAILS

	am	pm	front	back	other
_____	☐	☐			☐ Nausea
_____	☐	☐			☐ Diarrhea
_____	☐	☐			☐ Vomiting
_____	☐	☐			☐ Sore throat
_____	☐	☐			☐ Congestion
_____	☐	☐			☐ Coughing
_____	☐	☐			☐ Chills
_____	☐	☐			☐ Fever

SLEEP

hours　　　*quality*
_____　(1) (2) (3) (4) (5)

STRESS LEVELS

None	Low	Medium	High	Max	@$#%!

WEATHER

☐ Cold　☐ Mild　☐ Hot
☐ Dry　☐ Humid　☐ Wet
Allergen Levels: _____
BM Pressure: _____

EXERCISE

☐ Heck yes, I worked out.
☐ I managed to exercise a bit.
☐ No, I haven't exercised at all.
☐ I did some stuff, and that counts.

DETAILS

FOOD / MEDICATION

Food / Drinks

Meds / Supplements	Time	Dose

☐ usual daily medication

Notes
_____
_____

I am grateful for...
_____

HOW ARE YOU *Feeling today?*

😍 Amazing!	🙂 Meh
😁 Great	😠 Not good
🙂 Good	😣 Terrible!

RATE YOUR PAIN LEVEL

① ② ③ ④ ⑤ ⑥ ⑦ ⑧ ⑨ ⑩

WHAT ABOUT YOUR...?

Mood	① ② ③ ④ ⑤ ⑥ ⑦ ⑧ ⑨ ⑩
Energy Levels	① ② ③ ④ ⑤ ⑥ ⑦ ⑧ ⑨ ⑩
Mental Clarity	① ② ③ ④ ⑤ ⑥ ⑦ ⑧ ⑨ ⑩

PAIN & SYMPTOM DETAILS

	am	pm	*front*	*back*	*other*
_____	☐	☐			☐ Nausea
_____	☐	☐			☐ Diarrhea
_____	☐	☐			☐ Vomiting
_____	☐	☐			☐ Sore throat
_____	☐	☐			☐ Congestion
_____	☐	☐			☐ Coughing
_____	☐	☐			☐ Chills
_____	☐	☐			☐ Fever

SLEEP

hours
_____

quality
① ② ③ ④ ⑤

STRESS LEVELS

None	Low	Medium	High	Max	@$#%!

WEATHER

☐ Cold   ☐ Mild   ☐ Hot
☐ Dry   ☐ Humid   ☐ Wet

Allergen Levels: _____
BM Pressure: _____

EXERCISE

☐ Heck yes, I worked out.
☐ I managed to exercise a bit.
☐ No, I haven't exercised at all.
☐ I did some stuff, and that counts.

DETAILS

FOOD / MEDICATION

Food / Drinks

Meds / Supplements	Time	Dose

☐ usual daily medication

Notes
_____

I am grateful for...

HOW ARE YOU *Feeling today?*

😍 Amazing!	🙂 Meh
😁 Great	😠 Not good
😊 Good	😖 Terrible!

RATE YOUR PAIN LEVEL

① ② ③ ④ ⑤ ⑥ ⑦ ⑧ ⑨ ⑩

WHAT ABOUT YOUR...?

Mood	① ② ③ ④ ⑤ ⑥ ⑦ ⑧ ⑨ ⑩
Energy Levels	① ② ③ ④ ⑤ ⑥ ⑦ ⑧ ⑨ ⑩
Mental Clarity	① ② ③ ④ ⑤ ⑥ ⑦ ⑧ ⑨ ⑩

PAIN & SYMPTOM DETAILS

	am	pm	front	back	other
	☐	☐			☐ Nausea
	☐	☐			☐ Diarrhea
	☐	☐			☐ Vomiting
	☐	☐			☐ Sore throat
	☐	☐			☐ Congestion
	☐	☐			☐ Coughing
	☐	☐			☐ Chills
	☐	☐			☐ Fever

SLEEP

hours _____ *quality* ① ② ③ ④ ⑤

STRESS LEVELS

None	Low	Medium	High	Max	@$#%!

WEATHER

☐ Cold ☐ Mild ☐ Hot
☐ Dry ☐ Humid ☐ Wet
Allergen Levels: _____
BM Pressure: _____

EXERCISE

☐ Heck yes, I worked out.
☐ I managed to exercise a bit.
☐ No, I haven't exercised at all.
☐ I did some stuff, and that counts.

DETAILS

FOOD / MEDICATION

Food / Drinks

Meds / Supplements	Time	Dose

☐ usual daily medication

Notes

I am grateful for...

| M T W T F S S | DATE:

HOW ARE YOU *Feeling today?*

😍 Amazing!	🙂 Meh
😁 Great	😠 Not good
😊 Good	😖 Terrible!

RATE YOUR PAIN LEVEL

(1) (2) (3) (4) (5) (6) (7) (8) (9) (10)

WHAT ABOUT YOUR...?

Mood	(1) (2) (3) (4) (5) (6) (7) (8) (9) (10)
Energy Levels	(1) (2) (3) (4) (5) (6) (7) (8) (9) (10)
Mental Clarity	(1) (2) (3) (4) (5) (6) (7) (8) (9) (10)

PAIN & SYMPTOM DETAILS

	am	pm	*front*	*back*	*other*
_____	☐	☐			☐ Nausea
_____	☐	☐			☐ Diarrhea
_____	☐	☐			☐ Vomiting
_____	☐	☐			☐ Sore throat
_____	☐	☐			☐ Congestion
_____	☐	☐			☐ Coughing
_____	☐	☐			☐ Chills
_____	☐	☐			☐ Fever

SLEEP

hours
_____

quality
(1) (2) (3) (4) (5)

STRESS LEVELS

None	Low	Medium	High	Max	@$#%!

WEATHER

☐ Cold   ☐ Mild   ☐ Hot
☐ Dry   ☐ Humid   ☐ Wet
Allergen Levels: _____
BM Pressure: _____

EXERCISE

☐ Heck yes, I worked out.
☐ I managed to exercise a bit.
☐ No, I haven't exercised at all.
☐ I did some stuff, and that counts.

DETAILS

FOOD / MEDICATION

Food / Drinks

Meds / Supplements	Time	Dose

☐ usual daily medication

Notes
_____
_____

I am grateful for...

HOW ARE YOU *Feeling today?*

😍 Amazing!	🙂 Meh
😁 Great	😠 Not good
😊 Good	😖 Terrible!

RATE YOUR PAIN LEVEL

① ② ③ ④ ⑤ ⑥ ⑦ ⑧ ⑨ ⑩

WHAT ABOUT YOUR...?

Mood	① ② ③ ④ ⑤ ⑥ ⑦ ⑧ ⑨ ⑩
Energy Levels	① ② ③ ④ ⑤ ⑥ ⑦ ⑧ ⑨ ⑩
Mental Clarity	① ② ③ ④ ⑤ ⑥ ⑦ ⑧ ⑨ ⑩

PAIN & SYMPTOM DETAILS

	am	pm	front	back	other
	☐	☐			☐ Nausea
	☐	☐			☐ Diarrhea
	☐	☐			☐ Vomiting
	☐	☐			☐ Sore throat
	☐	☐			☐ Congestion
	☐	☐			☐ Coughing
	☐	☐			☐ Chills
	☐	☐			☐ Fever

SLEEP

hours _____   *quality* ① ② ③ ④ ⑤

STRESS LEVELS

None	Low	Medium	High	Max	@$#%!

WEATHER

☐ Cold   ☐ Mild   ☐ Hot
☐ Dry   ☐ Humid   ☐ Wet
Allergen Levels: _____
BM Pressure: _____

EXERCISE

☐ Heck yes, I worked out.
☐ I managed to exercise a bit.
☐ No, I haven't exercised at all.
☐ I did some stuff, and that counts.

DETAILS

FOOD / MEDICATION

Food / Drinks

Meds / Supplements	Time	Dose

☐ usual daily medication

Notes
_____
_____

I am grateful for...

M T W T F S S   DATE:

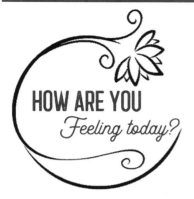

HOW ARE YOU *Feeling today?*

😍 Amazing!	🙂 Meh
😁 Great	😠 Not good
😊 Good	😣 Terrible!

RATE YOUR PAIN LEVEL

① ② ③ ④ ⑤ ⑥ ⑦ ⑧ ⑨ ⑩

WHAT ABOUT YOUR...?

Mood	① ② ③ ④ ⑤ ⑥ ⑦ ⑧ ⑨ ⑩
Energy Levels	① ② ③ ④ ⑤ ⑥ ⑦ ⑧ ⑨ ⑩
Mental Clarity	① ② ③ ④ ⑤ ⑥ ⑦ ⑧ ⑨ ⑩

PAIN & SYMPTOM DETAILS

	am	pm	*front*	*back*	*other*
_____	☐	☐			☐ Nausea
_____	☐	☐			☐ Diarrhea
_____	☐	☐			☐ Vomiting
_____	☐	☐			☐ Sore throat
_____	☐	☐			☐ Congestion
_____	☐	☐			☐ Coughing
_____	☐	☐			☐ Chills
_____	☐	☐			☐ Fever

SLEEP

hours _____   *quality* ① ② ③ ④ ⑤

STRESS LEVELS

None	Low	Medium	High	Max	@$#%!

WEATHER

☐ Cold   ☐ Mild   ☐ Hot
☐ Dry   ☐ Humid ☐ Wet
Allergen Levels: _____
BM Pressure: _____

EXERCISE

☐ Heck yes, I worked out.
☐ I managed to exercise a bit.
☐ No, I haven't exercised at all.
☐ I did some stuff, and that counts.

DETAILS

FOOD / MEDICATION

Food / Drinks

Meds / Supplements	Time	Dose

☐ usual daily medication

Notes
_____

I am grateful for...
_____

HOW ARE YOU Feeling today?

😍 Amazing!	🙂 Meh
😁 Great	😠 Not good
😊 Good	😖 Terrible!

RATE YOUR PAIN LEVEL

① ② ③ ④ ⑤ ⑥ ⑦ ⑧ ⑨ ⑩

WHAT ABOUT YOUR...?

Mood	① ② ③ ④ ⑤ ⑥ ⑦ ⑧ ⑨ ⑩
Energy Levels	① ② ③ ④ ⑤ ⑥ ⑦ ⑧ ⑨ ⑩
Mental Clarity	① ② ③ ④ ⑤ ⑥ ⑦ ⑧ ⑨ ⑩

PAIN & SYMPTOM DETAILS

	am	pm	front	back	other
_____	☐	☐			☐ Nausea
_____	☐	☐			☐ Diarrhea
_____	☐	☐			☐ Vomiting
_____	☐	☐			☐ Sore throat
_____	☐	☐			☐ Congestion
_____	☐	☐			☐ Coughing
_____	☐	☐			☐ Chills
_____	☐	☐			☐ Fever

SLEEP

hours _____

quality ① ② ③ ④ ⑤

STRESS LEVELS

None	Low	Medium	High	Max	@$#%!

WEATHER

☐ Cold   ☐ Mild   ☐ Hot
☐ Dry   ☐ Humid   ☐ Wet

Allergen Levels: _____
BM Pressure: _____

EXERCISE

☐ Heck yes, I worked out.
☐ I managed to exercise a bit.
☐ No, I haven't exercised at all.
☐ I did some stuff, and that counts.

DETAILS

FOOD / MEDICATION

Food / Drinks

Meds / Supplements	Time	Dose
☐ usual daily medication		

Notes
_____

I am grateful for...

M T W T F S S   DATE:

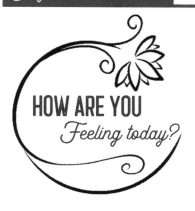

HOW ARE YOU *Feeling today?*

☺ Amazing!	☺ Meh
☺ Great	☹ Not good
☺ Good	☹ Terrible!

RATE YOUR PAIN LEVEL

① ② ③ ④ ⑤ ⑥ ⑦ ⑧ ⑨ ⑩

WHAT ABOUT YOUR...?

Mood	① ② ③ ④ ⑤ ⑥ ⑦ ⑧ ⑨ ⑩
Energy Levels	① ② ③ ④ ⑤ ⑥ ⑦ ⑧ ⑨ ⑩
Mental Clarity	① ② ③ ④ ⑤ ⑥ ⑦ ⑧ ⑨ ⑩

PAIN & SYMPTOM DETAILS

	am	pm	*front*	*back*	*other*
_____	☐	☐			☐ Nausea
_____	☐	☐			☐ Diarrhea
_____	☐	☐			☐ Vomiting
_____	☐	☐			☐ Sore throat
_____	☐	☐			☐ Congestion
_____	☐	☐			☐ Coughing
_____	☐	☐			☐ Chills
_____	☐	☐			☐ Fever

SLEEP

hours
_____

quality
① ② ③ ④ ⑤

STRESS LEVELS

None	Low	Medium	High	Max	@$#%!

WEATHER

☐ Cold   ☐ Mild   ☐ Hot
☐ Dry   ☐ Humid   ☐ Wet
Allergen Levels: _____
BM Pressure: _____

EXERCISE

☐ Heck yes, I worked out.
☐ I managed to exercise a bit.
☐ No, I haven't exercised at all.
☐ I did some stuff, and that counts.

DETAILS

FOOD / MEDICATION

Food / Drinks

Meds / Supplements	Time	Dose

☐ usual daily medication

Notes
_____

I am grateful for...
_____

HOW ARE YOU Feeling today?

😍 Amazing!	🙂 Meh
😁 Great	😣 Not good
😊 Good	😵 Terrible!

RATE YOUR PAIN LEVEL

1 2 3 4 5 6 7 8 9 10

WHAT ABOUT YOUR...?

Mood	1 2 3 4 5 6 7 8 9 10
Energy Levels	1 2 3 4 5 6 7 8 9 10
Mental Clarity	1 2 3 4 5 6 7 8 9 10

PAIN & SYMPTOM DETAILS

	am	pm	front	back	other
	☐	☐			☐ Nausea
	☐	☐			☐ Diarrhea
	☐	☐			☐ Vomiting
	☐	☐			☐ Sore throat
	☐	☐			☐ Congestion
	☐	☐			☐ Coughing
	☐	☐			☐ Chills
	☐	☐			☐ Fever

SLEEP

hours _____   quality 1 2 3 4 5

STRESS LEVELS

None	Low	Medium	High	Max	@$#%!

WEATHER

☐ Cold   ☐ Mild   ☐ Hot
☐ Dry   ☐ Humid   ☐ Wet

Allergen Levels: _____
BM Pressure: _____

EXERCISE

☐ Heck yes, I worked out.
☐ I managed to exercise a bit.
☐ No, I haven't exercised at all.
☐ I did some stuff, and that counts.

DETAILS

FOOD / MEDICATION

Food / Drinks

Meds / Supplements	Time	Dose

☐ usual daily medication

Notes
_____
_____

I am grateful for...
_____

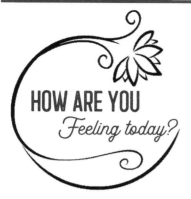

HOW ARE YOU *Feeling today?*

Amazing!	Meh
Great	Not good
Good	Terrible!

RATE YOUR PAIN LEVEL

① ② ③ ④ ⑤ ⑥ ⑦ ⑧ ⑨ ⑩

WHAT ABOUT YOUR...?

Mood	① ② ③ ④ ⑤ ⑥ ⑦ ⑧ ⑨ ⑩
Energy Levels	① ② ③ ④ ⑤ ⑥ ⑦ ⑧ ⑨ ⑩
Mental Clarity	① ② ③ ④ ⑤ ⑥ ⑦ ⑧ ⑨ ⑩

PAIN & SYMPTOM DETAILS

	am	pm	*front*	*back*	*other*
	☐	☐			☐ Nausea
	☐	☐			☐ Diarrhea
	☐	☐			☐ Vomiting
	☐	☐			☐ Sore throat
	☐	☐			☐ Congestion
	☐	☐			☐ Coughing
	☐	☐			☐ Chills
	☐	☐			☐ Fever

SLEEP

hours
_____

quality
① ② ③ ④ ⑤

STRESS LEVELS

None	Low	Medium	High	Max	@$#%!

WEATHER

☐ Cold ☐ Mild ☐ Hot
☐ Dry ☐ Humid ☐ Wet
Allergen Levels: _____
BM Pressure: _____

EXERCISE

☐ Heck yes, I worked out.
☐ I managed to exercise a bit.
☐ No, I haven't exercised at all.
☐ I did some stuff, and that counts.

DETAILS

FOOD / MEDICATION

Food / Drinks	Meds / Supplements	Time	Dose
	☐ usual daily medication		

Notes

I am grateful for...

HOW ARE YOU Feeling today?

Amazing!	Meh
Great	Not good
Good	Terrible!

RATE YOUR PAIN LEVEL

1 2 3 4 5 6 7 8 9 10

WHAT ABOUT YOUR...?

Mood	1 2 3 4 5 6 7 8 9 10
Energy Levels	1 2 3 4 5 6 7 8 9 10
Mental Clarity	1 2 3 4 5 6 7 8 9 10

PAIN & SYMPTOM DETAILS

	am	pm	front	back	other
_____	☐	☐			☐ Nausea
_____	☐	☐			☐ Diarrhea
_____	☐	☐			☐ Vomiting
_____	☐	☐			☐ Sore throat
_____	☐	☐			☐ Congestion
_____	☐	☐			☐ Coughing
_____	☐	☐			☐ Chills
_____	☐	☐			☐ Fever

SLEEP

hours
_____

quality
1 2 3 4 5

STRESS LEVELS

None	Low	Medium	High	Max	@$#%!

WEATHER

☐ Cold   ☐ Mild   ☐ Hot
☐ Dry   ☐ Humid   ☐ Wet

Allergen Levels: _____
BM Pressure: _____

EXERCISE

☐ Heck yes, I worked out.
☐ I managed to exercise a bit.
☐ No, I haven't exercised at all.
☐ I did some stuff, and that counts.

DETAILS

FOOD / MEDICATION

Food / Drinks

Meds / Supplements	Time	Dose

☐ usual daily medication

Notes
_____
_____

I am grateful for...

HOW ARE YOU *Feeling today?*

Amazing!	Meh
Great	Not good
Good	Terrible!

RATE YOUR PAIN LEVEL

① ② ③ ④ ⑤ ⑥ ⑦ ⑧ ⑨ ⑩

WHAT ABOUT YOUR...?

Mood	① ② ③ ④ ⑤ ⑥ ⑦ ⑧ ⑨ ⑩
Energy Levels	① ② ③ ④ ⑤ ⑥ ⑦ ⑧ ⑨ ⑩
Mental Clarity	① ② ③ ④ ⑤ ⑥ ⑦ ⑧ ⑨ ⑩

PAIN & SYMPTOM DETAILS

	am	pm	*front*	*back*	*other*
	☐	☐			☐ Nausea
	☐	☐			☐ Diarrhea
	☐	☐			☐ Vomiting
	☐	☐			☐ Sore throat
	☐	☐			☐ Congestion
	☐	☐			☐ Coughing
	☐	☐			☐ Chills
	☐	☐			☐ Fever

SLEEP

hours _____

quality ① ② ③ ④ ⑤

STRESS LEVELS

None	Low	Medium	High	Max	@$#%!

WEATHER

☐ Cold   ☐ Mild   ☐ Hot
☐ Dry   ☐ Humid ☐ Wet

Allergen Levels: _____
BM Pressure: _____

EXERCISE

☐ Heck yes, I worked out.
☐ I managed to exercise a bit.
☐ No, I haven't exercised at all.
☐ I did some stuff, and that counts.

DETAILS

FOOD / MEDICATION

Food / Drinks

Meds / Supplements	Time	Dose

☐ usual daily medication

Notes

I am grateful for...

M T W T F S S   DATE:

HOW ARE YOU Feeling today?

Amazing!	Meh
Great	Not good
Good	Terrible!

RATE YOUR PAIN LEVEL

① ② ③ ④ ⑤ ⑥ ⑦ ⑧ ⑨ ⑩

WHAT ABOUT YOUR...?

Mood	① ② ③ ④ ⑤ ⑥ ⑦ ⑧ ⑨ ⑩
Energy Levels	① ② ③ ④ ⑤ ⑥ ⑦ ⑧ ⑨ ⑩
Mental Clarity	① ② ③ ④ ⑤ ⑥ ⑦ ⑧ ⑨ ⑩

PAIN & SYMPTOM DETAILS

	am	pm	*front*	*back*	*other*
_____	☐	☐			☐ Nausea
_____	☐	☐			☐ Diarrhea
_____	☐	☐			☐ Vomiting
_____	☐	☐			☐ Sore throat
_____	☐	☐			☐ Congestion
_____	☐	☐			☐ Coughing
_____	☐	☐			☐ Chills
_____	☐	☐			☐ Fever

SLEEP

hours
_____

quality
① ② ③ ④ ⑤

STRESS LEVELS

None	Low	Medium	High	Max	@$#%!

WEATHER

☐ Cold   ☐ Mild   ☐ Hot
☐ Dry   ☐ Humid   ☐ Wet

Allergen Levels: _____
BM Pressure: _____

EXERCISE

☐ Heck yes, I worked out.
☐ I managed to exercise a bit.
☐ No, I haven't exercised at all.
☐ I did some stuff, and that counts.

DETAILS

FOOD / MEDICATION

Food / Drinks

Meds / Supplements	Time	Dose

☐ usual daily medication

Notes
_____
_____

I am grateful for...
_____

M T W T F S S   DATE:

HOW ARE YOU
Feeling today?

Amazing!	Meh
Great	Not good
Good	Terrible!

RATE YOUR PAIN LEVEL

① ② ③ ④ ⑤ ⑥ ⑦ ⑧ ⑨ ⑩

WHAT ABOUT YOUR...?

Mood	① ② ③ ④ ⑤ ⑥ ⑦ ⑧ ⑨ ⑩
Energy Levels	① ② ③ ④ ⑤ ⑥ ⑦ ⑧ ⑨ ⑩
Mental Clarity	① ② ③ ④ ⑤ ⑥ ⑦ ⑧ ⑨ ⑩

PAIN & SYMPTOM DETAILS

	am	pm	*front*	*back*	*other*
_____	☐	☐			☐ Nausea
_____	☐	☐			☐ Diarrhea
_____	☐	☐			☐ Vomiting
_____	☐	☐			☐ Sore throat
_____	☐	☐			☐ Congestion
_____	☐	☐			☐ Coughing
_____	☐	☐			☐ Chills
_____	☐	☐			☐ Fever

SLEEP

hours   *quality*
_____   ① ② ③ ④ ⑤

STRESS LEVELS

None	Low	Medium	High	Max	@$#%!

WEATHER

☐ Cold   ☐ Mild   ☐ Hot
☐ Dry   ☐ Humid   ☐ Wet
Allergen Levels: _____
BM Pressure: _____

EXERCISE

☐ Heck yes, I worked out.
☐ I managed to exercise a bit.
☐ No, I haven't exercised at all.
☐ I did some stuff, and that counts.

DETAILS

FOOD / MEDICATION

Food / Drinks

Meds / Supplements	Time	Dose

☐ usual daily medication

Notes
_____
_____

I am grateful for...

HOW ARE YOU *Feeling today?*

😍 Amazing!	🙂 Meh
😁 Great	😠 Not good
😊 Good	😖 Terrible!

RATE YOUR PAIN LEVEL

① ② ③ ④ ⑤ ⑥ ⑦ ⑧ ⑨ ⑩

WHAT ABOUT YOUR...?

Mood	① ② ③ ④ ⑤ ⑥ ⑦ ⑧ ⑨ ⑩
Energy Levels	① ② ③ ④ ⑤ ⑥ ⑦ ⑧ ⑨ ⑩
Mental Clarity	① ② ③ ④ ⑤ ⑥ ⑦ ⑧ ⑨ ⑩

PAIN & SYMPTOM DETAILS

	am	pm	*front*	*back*	*other*
_____	☐	☐			☐ Nausea
_____	☐	☐			☐ Diarrhea
_____	☐	☐			☐ Vomiting
_____	☐	☐			☐ Sore throat
_____	☐	☐			☐ Congestion
_____	☐	☐			☐ Coughing
_____	☐	☐			☐ Chills
_____	☐	☐			☐ Fever

SLEEP

hours _____   *quality* ① ② ③ ④ ⑤

STRESS LEVELS

None	Low	Medium	High	Max	@$#%!

WEATHER

☐ Cold   ☐ Mild   ☐ Hot
☐ Dry   ☐ Humid   ☐ Wet
Allergen Levels: _____
BM Pressure: _____

EXERCISE

☐ Heck yes, I worked out.
☐ I managed to exercise a bit.
☐ No, I haven't exercised at all.
☐ I did some stuff, and that counts.

DETAILS

FOOD / MEDICATION

Food / Drinks	Meds / Supplements	Time	Dose

☐ usual daily medication

Notes
_____
_____

I am grateful for...

HOW ARE YOU *Feeling today?*

😍 Amazing!	🙂 Meh
😁 Great	😠 Not good
😊 Good	😤 Terrible!

RATE YOUR PAIN LEVEL

① ② ③ ④ ⑤ ⑥ ⑦ ⑧ ⑨ ⑩

WHAT ABOUT YOUR...?

Mood	① ② ③ ④ ⑤ ⑥ ⑦ ⑧ ⑨ ⑩
Energy Levels	① ② ③ ④ ⑤ ⑥ ⑦ ⑧ ⑨ ⑩
Mental Clarity	① ② ③ ④ ⑤ ⑥ ⑦ ⑧ ⑨ ⑩

PAIN & SYMPTOM DETAILS

	am	pm	*front*	*back*	*other*
_____	☐	☐			☐ Nausea
_____	☐	☐			☐ Diarrhea
_____	☐	☐			☐ Vomiting
_____	☐	☐			☐ Sore throat
_____	☐	☐			☐ Congestion
_____	☐	☐			☐ Coughing
_____	☐	☐			☐ Chills
_____	☐	☐			☐ Fever

SLEEP

hours
_____

quality
① ② ③ ④ ⑤

STRESS LEVELS

None	Low	Medium	High	Max	@$#%!

WEATHER

☐ Cold   ☐ Mild   ☐ Hot
☐ Dry   ☐ Humid   ☐ Wet

Allergen Levels: _____
BM Pressure: _____

EXERCISE

☐ Heck yes, I worked out.
☐ I managed to exercise a bit.
☐ No, I haven't exercised at all.
☐ I did some stuff, and that counts.

DETAILS

FOOD / MEDICATION

Food / Drinks

Meds / Supplements	Time	Dose

☐ usual daily medication

Notes
_____
_____

I am grateful for...

HOW ARE YOU *Feeling today?*

Amazing!	Meh
Great	Not good
Good	Terrible!

RATE YOUR PAIN LEVEL

① ② ③ ④ ⑤ ⑥ ⑦ ⑧ ⑨ ⑩

WHAT ABOUT YOUR...?

Mood	① ② ③ ④ ⑤ ⑥ ⑦ ⑧ ⑨ ⑩
Energy Levels	① ② ③ ④ ⑤ ⑥ ⑦ ⑧ ⑨ ⑩
Mental Clarity	① ② ③ ④ ⑤ ⑥ ⑦ ⑧ ⑨ ⑩

PAIN & SYMPTOM DETAILS

	am	pm	*front*	*back*	other
_____	☐	☐			☐ Nausea
_____	☐	☐			☐ Diarrhea
_____	☐	☐			☐ Vomiting
_____	☐	☐			☐ Sore throat
_____	☐	☐			☐ Congestion
_____	☐	☐			☐ Coughing
_____	☐	☐			☐ Chills
_____	☐	☐			☐ Fever

SLEEP

hours
_____

quality
① ② ③ ④ ⑤

STRESS LEVELS

None	Low	Medium	High	Max	@$#%!

WEATHER

☐ Cold   ☐ Mild   ☐ Hot
☐ Dry   ☐ Humid   ☐ Wet

Allergen Levels: _____
BM Pressure: _____

EXERCISE

☐ Heck yes, I worked out.
☐ I managed to exercise a bit.
☐ No, I haven't exercised at all.
☐ I did some stuff, and that counts.

DETAILS

FOOD / MEDICATION

Food / Drinks	Meds / Supplements	Time	Dose

☐ usual daily medication

Notes

I am grateful for...

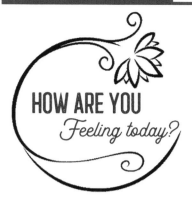

HOW ARE YOU *Feeling today?*

😍 Amazing!	🙂 Meh
😁 Great	😠 Not good
🙂 Good	😫 Terrible!

RATE YOUR PAIN LEVEL

① ② ③ ④ ⑤ ⑥ ⑦ ⑧ ⑨ ⑩

WHAT ABOUT YOUR...?

Mood	① ② ③ ④ ⑤ ⑥ ⑦ ⑧ ⑨ ⑩
Energy Levels	① ② ③ ④ ⑤ ⑥ ⑦ ⑧ ⑨ ⑩
Mental Clarity	① ② ③ ④ ⑤ ⑥ ⑦ ⑧ ⑨ ⑩

PAIN & SYMPTOM DETAILS

	am	pm	*front*	*back*	*other*
_____	☐	☐			☐ Nausea
_____	☐	☐			☐ Diarrhea
_____	☐	☐			☐ Vomiting
_____	☐	☐			☐ Sore throat
_____	☐	☐			☐ Congestion
_____	☐	☐			☐ Coughing
_____	☐	☐			☐ Chills
_____	☐	☐			☐ Fever

SLEEP

hours
_____

quality
① ② ③ ④ ⑤

STRESS LEVELS

None	Low	Medium	High	Max	@$#%!

WEATHER

☐ Cold   ☐ Mild   ☐ Hot
☐ Dry   ☐ Humid   ☐ Wet

Allergen Levels: _____
BM Pressure: _____

EXERCISE

☐ Heck yes, I worked out.
☐ I managed to exercise a bit.
☐ No, I haven't exercised at all.
☐ I did some stuff, and that counts.

DETAILS

FOOD / MEDICATION

Food / Drinks

Meds / Supplements	Time	Dose

☐ usual daily medication

Notes
_____

I am grateful for...
_____

M T W T F S S   DATE:

HOW ARE YOU *Feeling today?*

😍 Amazing!	🙂 Meh
😁 Great	😣 Not good
😊 Good	😵 Terrible!

RATE YOUR PAIN LEVEL

① ② ③ ④ ⑤ ⑥ ⑦ ⑧ ⑨ ⑩

WHAT ABOUT YOUR...?

Mood	① ② ③ ④ ⑤ ⑥ ⑦ ⑧ ⑨ ⑩
Energy Levels	① ② ③ ④ ⑤ ⑥ ⑦ ⑧ ⑨ ⑩
Mental Clarity	① ② ③ ④ ⑤ ⑥ ⑦ ⑧ ⑨ ⑩

PAIN & SYMPTOM DETAILS

	am	pm	*front*	*back*	*other*
_____	☐	☐			☐ Nausea
_____	☐	☐			☐ Diarrhea
_____	☐	☐			☐ Vomiting
_____	☐	☐			☐ Sore throat
_____	☐	☐			☐ Congestion
_____	☐	☐			☐ Coughing
_____	☐	☐			☐ Chills
_____	☐	☐			☐ Fever

SLEEP

hours   *quality*
_____   ① ② ③ ④ ⑤

STRESS LEVELS

None	Low	Medium	High	Max	@$#%!

WEATHER

☐ Cold   ☐ Mild   ☐ Hot
☐ Dry   ☐ Humid   ☐ Wet
Allergen Levels: _____
BM Pressure: _____

EXERCISE

☐ Heck yes, I worked out.
☐ I managed to exercise a bit.
☐ No, I haven't exercised at all.
☐ I did some stuff, and that counts.

DETAILS

FOOD / MEDICATION

Food / Drinks

Meds / Supplements	Time	Dose

☐ usual daily medication

Notes
_____
_____

I am grateful for...

HOW ARE YOU *Feeling today?*

😍 Amazing!	🙂 Meh
😁 Great	😠 Not good
🙂 Good	😖 Terrible!

RATE YOUR PAIN LEVEL

① ② ③ ④ ⑤ ⑥ ⑦ ⑧ ⑨ ⑩

WHAT ABOUT YOUR...?

Mood	① ② ③ ④ ⑤ ⑥ ⑦ ⑧ ⑨ ⑩
Energy Levels	① ② ③ ④ ⑤ ⑥ ⑦ ⑧ ⑨ ⑩
Mental Clarity	① ② ③ ④ ⑤ ⑥ ⑦ ⑧ ⑨ ⑩

PAIN & SYMPTOM DETAILS

	am	pm	*front*	*back*	*other*
_____	☐	☐			☐ Nausea
_____	☐	☐			☐ Diarrhea
_____	☐	☐			☐ Vomiting
_____	☐	☐			☐ Sore throat
_____	☐	☐			☐ Congestion
_____	☐	☐			☐ Coughing
_____	☐	☐			☐ Chills
_____	☐	☐			☐ Fever

SLEEP

hours
_____

quality
① ② ③ ④ ⑤

STRESS LEVELS

None	Low	Medium	High	Max	@$#%!

WEATHER

☐ Cold   ☐ Mild   ☐ Hot
☐ Dry   ☐ Humid   ☐ Wet
Allergen Levels: _____
BM Pressure: _____

EXERCISE

☐ Heck yes, I worked out.
☐ I managed to exercise a bit.
☐ No, I haven't exercised at all.
☐ I did some stuff, and that counts.

DETAILS

FOOD / MEDICATION

Food / Drinks

Meds / Supplements	Time	Dose

☐ usual daily medication

Notes
_____
_____

I am grateful for...
_____

HOW ARE YOU Feeling today?

😍 Amazing!	🙂 Meh
😁 Great	😣 Not good
😊 Good	😵 Terrible!

RATE YOUR PAIN LEVEL

(1) (2) (3) (4) (5) (6) (7) (8) (9) (10)

WHAT ABOUT YOUR...?

Mood	(1) (2) (3) (4) (5) (6) (7) (8) (9) (10)
Energy Levels	(1) (2) (3) (4) (5) (6) (7) (8) (9) (10)
Mental Clarity	(1) (2) (3) (4) (5) (6) (7) (8) (9) (10)

PAIN & SYMPTOM DETAILS

	am	pm	front	back	other
_____	☐	☐			☐ Nausea
_____	☐	☐			☐ Diarrhea
_____	☐	☐			☐ Vomiting
_____	☐	☐			☐ Sore throat
_____	☐	☐			☐ Congestion
_____	☐	☐			☐ Coughing
_____	☐	☐			☐ Chills
_____	☐	☐			☐ Fever

SLEEP

hours _____   _quality_ (1) (2) (3) (4) (5)

STRESS LEVELS

None	Low	Medium	High	Max	@$#%!

WEATHER

☐ Cold   ☐ Mild   ☐ Hot
☐ Dry   ☐ Humid   ☐ Wet
Allergen Levels: _____
BM Pressure: _____

EXERCISE

☐ Heck yes, I worked out.
☐ I managed to exercise a bit.
☐ No, I haven't exercised at all.
☐ I did some stuff, and that counts.

DETAILS

FOOD / MEDICATION

Food / Drinks

Meds / Supplements	Time	Dose

☐ usual daily medication

Notes
_____

I am grateful for...

M T W T F S S   DATE:

HOW ARE YOU *Feeling today?*

☺ Amazing!	☺ Meh
☺ Great	☹ Not good
☺ Good	☹ Terrible!

RATE YOUR PAIN LEVEL

① ② ③ ④ ⑤ ⑥ ⑦ ⑧ ⑨ ⑩

WHAT ABOUT YOUR...?

Mood	① ② ③ ④ ⑤ ⑥ ⑦ ⑧ ⑨ ⑩
Energy Levels	① ② ③ ④ ⑤ ⑥ ⑦ ⑧ ⑨ ⑩
Mental Clarity	① ② ③ ④ ⑤ ⑥ ⑦ ⑧ ⑨ ⑩

PAIN & SYMPTOM DETAILS

	am	pm	*front*	*back*	*other*
_____	☐	☐			☐ Nausea
_____	☐	☐			☐ Diarrhea
_____	☐	☐			☐ Vomiting
_____	☐	☐			☐ Sore throat
_____	☐	☐			☐ Congestion
_____	☐	☐			☐ Coughing
_____	☐	☐			☐ Chills
_____	☐	☐			☐ Fever

SLEEP

hours _____

quality ① ② ③ ④ ⑤

STRESS LEVELS

None	Low	Medium	High	Max	@$#%!

WEATHER

☐ Cold ☐ Mild ☐ Hot
☐ Dry ☐ Humid ☐ Wet
Allergen Levels: _____
BM Pressure: _____

EXERCISE

☐ Heck yes, I worked out.
☐ I managed to exercise a bit.
☐ No, I haven't exercised at all.
☐ I did some stuff, and that counts.

DETAILS

FOOD / MEDICATION

Food / Drinks		Meds / Supplements	Time	Dose
		☐ usual daily medication		

Notes

_____

I am grateful for...

HOW ARE YOU Feeling today?

😍 Amazing!	🙂 Meh
😁 Great	😣 Not good
😊 Good	😖 Terrible!

RATE YOUR PAIN LEVEL

① ② ③ ④ ⑤ ⑥ ⑦ ⑧ ⑨ ⑩

WHAT ABOUT YOUR...?

Mood	① ② ③ ④ ⑤ ⑥ ⑦ ⑧ ⑨ ⑩
Energy Levels	① ② ③ ④ ⑤ ⑥ ⑦ ⑧ ⑨ ⑩
Mental Clarity	① ② ③ ④ ⑤ ⑥ ⑦ ⑧ ⑨ ⑩

PAIN & SYMPTOM DETAILS

	am	pm	front	back	other
_____	☐	☐			☐ Nausea
_____	☐	☐			☐ Diarrhea
_____	☐	☐			☐ Vomiting
_____	☐	☐			☐ Sore throat
_____	☐	☐			☐ Congestion
_____	☐	☐			☐ Coughing
_____	☐	☐			☐ Chills
_____	☐	☐			☐ Fever

SLEEP

hours _____ quality ① ② ③ ④ ⑤

STRESS LEVELS

None	Low	Medium	High	Max	@$#%!

WEATHER

☐ Cold   ☐ Mild   ☐ Hot
☐ Dry   ☐ Humid ☐ Wet
Allergen Levels: _____
BM Pressure: _____

EXERCISE

☐ Heck yes, I worked out.
☐ I managed to exercise a bit.
☐ No, I haven't exercised at all.
☐ I did some stuff, and that counts.

DETAILS

FOOD / MEDICATION

Food / Drinks	Meds / Supplements	Time	Dose
	☐ usual daily medication		

Notes
_____
_____

I am grateful for...
_____

M T W T F S S   DATE:

HOW ARE YOU *Feeling today?*

Amazing!	Meh
Great	Not good
Good	Terrible!

RATE YOUR PAIN LEVEL

① ② ③ ④ ⑤ ⑥ ⑦ ⑧ ⑨ ⑩

WHAT ABOUT YOUR...?

Mood	① ② ③ ④ ⑤ ⑥ ⑦ ⑧ ⑨ ⑩
Energy Levels	① ② ③ ④ ⑤ ⑥ ⑦ ⑧ ⑨ ⑩
Mental Clarity	① ② ③ ④ ⑤ ⑥ ⑦ ⑧ ⑨ ⑩

PAIN & SYMPTOM DETAILS

	am	pm	*front*	*back*	*other*
	☐	☐			☐ Nausea
	☐	☐			☐ Diarrhea
	☐	☐			☐ Vomiting
	☐	☐			☐ Sore throat
	☐	☐			☐ Congestion
	☐	☐			☐ Coughing
	☐	☐			☐ Chills
	☐	☐			☐ Fever

SLEEP

hours
_____

quality
① ② ③ ④ ⑤

STRESS LEVELS

None	Low	Medium	High	Max	@$#%!

WEATHER

☐ Cold   ☐ Mild   ☐ Hot
☐ Dry   ☐ Humid   ☐ Wet

Allergen Levels: _____
BM Pressure: _____

EXERCISE

☐ Heck yes, I worked out.
☐ I managed to exercise a bit.
☐ No, I haven't exercised at all.
☐ I did some stuff, and that counts.

DETAILS

FOOD / MEDICATION

Food / Drinks

Meds / Supplements	Time	Dose

☐ usual daily medication

Notes

I am grateful for...

HOW ARE YOU Feeling today?

😍 Amazing!	🙂 Meh
😁 Great	😠 Not good
😊 Good	😖 Terrible!

RATE YOUR PAIN LEVEL

① ② ③ ④ ⑤ ⑥ ⑦ ⑧ ⑨ ⑩

WHAT ABOUT YOUR...?

Mood	① ② ③ ④ ⑤ ⑥ ⑦ ⑧ ⑨ ⑩
Energy Levels	① ② ③ ④ ⑤ ⑥ ⑦ ⑧ ⑨ ⑩
Mental Clarity	① ② ③ ④ ⑤ ⑥ ⑦ ⑧ ⑨ ⑩

PAIN & SYMPTOM DETAILS

	am	pm	front	back	other
_____	☐	☐			☐ Nausea
_____	☐	☐			☐ Diarrhea
_____	☐	☐			☐ Vomiting
_____	☐	☐			☐ Sore throat
_____	☐	☐			☐ Congestion
_____	☐	☐			☐ Coughing
_____	☐	☐			☐ Chills
_____	☐	☐			☐ Fever

SLEEP

hours _____   quality ① ② ③ ④ ⑤

STRESS LEVELS

None	Low	Medium	High	Max	@$#%!

WEATHER

☐ Cold   ☐ Mild   ☐ Hot
☐ Dry   ☐ Humid ☐ Wet
Allergen Levels: _____
BM Pressure: _____

EXERCISE

☐ Heck yes, I worked out.
☐ I managed to exercise a bit.
☐ No, I haven't exercised at all.
☐ I did some stuff, and that counts.

DETAILS

FOOD / MEDICATION

Food / Drinks

Meds / Supplements	Time	Dose

☐ usual daily medication

Notes
_____

I am grateful for...

M T W T F S S

DATE:

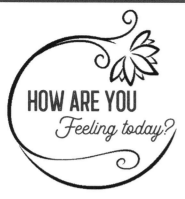

HOW ARE YOU *Feeling today?*

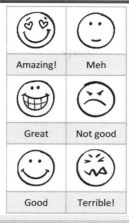

Amazing!	Meh
Great	Not good
Good	Terrible!

RATE YOUR PAIN LEVEL

① ② ③ ④ ⑤ ⑥ ⑦ ⑧ ⑨ ⑩

WHAT ABOUT YOUR...?

Mood	① ② ③ ④ ⑤ ⑥ ⑦ ⑧ ⑨ ⑩
Energy Levels	① ② ③ ④ ⑤ ⑥ ⑦ ⑧ ⑨ ⑩
Mental Clarity	① ② ③ ④ ⑤ ⑥ ⑦ ⑧ ⑨ ⑩

PAIN & SYMPTOM DETAILS

	am	pm	*front*	*back*	*other*
	☐	☐			☐ Nausea
	☐	☐			☐ Diarrhea
	☐	☐			☐ Vomiting
	☐	☐			☐ Sore throat
	☐	☐			☐ Congestion
	☐	☐			☐ Coughing
	☐	☐			☐ Chills
	☐	☐			☐ Fever

SLEEP

hours
_____

quality
① ② ③ ④ ⑤

STRESS LEVELS

None	Low	Medium	High	Max	@$#%!

WEATHER

☐ Cold ☐ Mild ☐ Hot
☐ Dry ☐ Humid ☐ Wet
Allergen Levels: _____
BM Pressure: _____

EXERCISE

☐ Heck yes, I worked out.
☐ I managed to exercise a bit.
☐ No, I haven't exercised at all.
☐ I did some stuff, and that counts.

DETAILS

FOOD / MEDICATION

Food / Drinks

Meds / Supplements	Time	Dose

☐ usual daily medication

Notes

_____

I am grateful for...

HOW ARE YOU *Feeling today?*

😍 Amazing!	🙂 Meh
😁 Great	😠 Not good
😊 Good	😫 Terrible!

RATE YOUR PAIN LEVEL

① ② ③ ④ ⑤ ⑥ ⑦ ⑧ ⑨ ⑩

WHAT ABOUT YOUR...?

Mood	① ② ③ ④ ⑤ ⑥ ⑦ ⑧ ⑨ ⑩
Energy Levels	① ② ③ ④ ⑤ ⑥ ⑦ ⑧ ⑨ ⑩
Mental Clarity	① ② ③ ④ ⑤ ⑥ ⑦ ⑧ ⑨ ⑩

PAIN & SYMPTOM DETAILS

	am	pm	front	back	other
_____	☐	☐			☐ Nausea
_____	☐	☐			☐ Diarrhea
_____	☐	☐			☐ Vomiting
_____	☐	☐			☐ Sore throat
_____	☐	☐			☐ Congestion
_____	☐	☐			☐ Coughing
_____	☐	☐			☐ Chills
_____	☐	☐			☐ Fever

SLEEP

hours
_____

quality
① ② ③ ④ ⑤

STRESS LEVELS

None	Low	Medium	High	Max	@$#%!

WEATHER

☐ Cold   ☐ Mild   ☐ Hot
☐ Dry   ☐ Humid   ☐ Wet

Allergen Levels: _____
BM Pressure: _____

EXERCISE

☐ Heck yes, I worked out.
☐ I managed to exercise a bit.
☐ No, I haven't exercised at all.
☐ I did some stuff, and that counts.

DETAILS

FOOD / MEDICATION

Food / Drinks

Meds / Supplements	Time	Dose

☐ usual daily medication

Notes
_____
_____

I am grateful for...
_____

M T W T F S S   DATE:

HOW ARE YOU *Feeling today?*

Amazing!	Meh
Great	Not good
Good	Terrible!

RATE YOUR PAIN LEVEL

(1) (2) (3) (4) (5) (6) (7) (8) (9) (10)

WHAT ABOUT YOUR...?

Mood	(1) (2) (3) (4) (5) (6) (7) (8) (9) (10)
Energy Levels	(1) (2) (3) (4) (5) (6) (7) (8) (9) (10)
Mental Clarity	(1) (2) (3) (4) (5) (6) (7) (8) (9) (10)

PAIN & SYMPTOM DETAILS

	am	pm	*front*	*back*	*other*
	☐	☐			☐ Nausea
	☐	☐			☐ Diarrhea
	☐	☐			☐ Vomiting
	☐	☐			☐ Sore throat
	☐	☐			☐ Congestion
	☐	☐			☐ Coughing
	☐	☐			☐ Chills
	☐	☐			☐ Fever

SLEEP

hours _____   *quality* (1) (2) (3) (4) (5)

STRESS LEVELS

None	Low	Medium	High	Max	@$#%!

WEATHER

☐ Cold   ☐ Mild   ☐ Hot
☐ Dry   ☐ Humid   ☐ Wet

Allergen Levels: _____
BM Pressure: _____

EXERCISE

☐ Heck yes, I worked out.
☐ I managed to exercise a bit.
☐ No, I haven't exercised at all.
☐ I did some stuff, and that counts.

DETAILS

FOOD / MEDICATION

Food / Drinks

Meds / Supplements	Time	Dose

☐ usual daily medication

Notes

I am grateful for…

HOW ARE YOU *Feeling today?*

😍 Amazing!	🙂 Meh
😁 Great	😠 Not good
😊 Good	😖 Terrible!

RATE YOUR PAIN LEVEL

① ② ③ ④ ⑤ ⑥ ⑦ ⑧ ⑨ ⑩

WHAT ABOUT YOUR...?

Mood	① ② ③ ④ ⑤ ⑥ ⑦ ⑧ ⑨ ⑩
Energy Levels	① ② ③ ④ ⑤ ⑥ ⑦ ⑧ ⑨ ⑩
Mental Clarity	① ② ③ ④ ⑤ ⑥ ⑦ ⑧ ⑨ ⑩

PAIN & SYMPTOM DETAILS

	am	pm	front	back	other
_____	☐	☐			☐ Nausea
_____	☐	☐			☐ Diarrhea
_____	☐	☐			☐ Vomiting
_____	☐	☐			☐ Sore throat
_____	☐	☐			☐ Congestion
_____	☐	☐			☐ Coughing
_____	☐	☐			☐ Chills
_____	☐	☐			☐ Fever

SLEEP

hours
_____

quality
① ② ③ ④ ⑤

STRESS LEVELS

None	Low	Medium	High	Max	@$#%!

WEATHER

☐ Cold ☐ Mild ☐ Hot
☐ Dry ☐ Humid ☐ Wet

Allergen Levels: _____
BM Pressure: _____

EXERCISE

☐ Heck yes, I worked out.
☐ I managed to exercise a bit.
☐ No, I haven't exercised at all.
☐ I did some stuff, and that counts.

DETAILS

FOOD / MEDICATION

Food / Drinks

Meds / Supplements	Time	Dose

☐ usual daily medication

Notes
_____
_____

I am grateful for...

HOW ARE YOU *Feeling today?*

😍 Amazing!	🙂 Meh
😁 Great	😠 Not good
🙂 Good	😖 Terrible!

RATE YOUR PAIN LEVEL

① ② ③ ④ ⑤ ⑥ ⑦ ⑧ ⑨ ⑩

WHAT ABOUT YOUR...?

Mood	① ② ③ ④ ⑤ ⑥ ⑦ ⑧ ⑨ ⑩
Energy Levels	① ② ③ ④ ⑤ ⑥ ⑦ ⑧ ⑨ ⑩
Mental Clarity	① ② ③ ④ ⑤ ⑥ ⑦ ⑧ ⑨ ⑩

PAIN & SYMPTOM DETAILS

	am	pm	*front*	*back*	*other*
	☐	☐			☐ Nausea
	☐	☐			☐ Diarrhea
	☐	☐			☐ Vomiting
	☐	☐			☐ Sore throat
	☐	☐			☐ Congestion
	☐	☐			☐ Coughing
	☐	☐			☐ Chills
	☐	☐			☐ Fever

SLEEP

hours _____

quality ① ② ③ ④ ⑤

STRESS LEVELS

None	Low	Medium	High	Max	@$#%!

WEATHER

☐ Cold   ☐ Mild   ☐ Hot
☐ Dry   ☐ Humid   ☐ Wet
Allergen Levels: _____
BM Pressure: _____

EXERCISE

☐ Heck yes, I worked out.
☐ I managed to exercise a bit.
☐ No, I haven't exercised at all.
☐ I did some stuff, and that counts.

DETAILS

FOOD / MEDICATION

Food / Drinks	Meds / Supplements	Time	Dose

☐ usual daily medication

Notes

I am grateful for…

HOW ARE YOU Feeling today?

Amazing!	Meh
Great	Not good
Good	Terrible!

RATE YOUR PAIN LEVEL

① ② ③ ④ ⑤ ⑥ ⑦ ⑧ ⑨ ⑩

WHAT ABOUT YOUR...?

Mood	① ② ③ ④ ⑤ ⑥ ⑦ ⑧ ⑨ ⑩
Energy Levels	① ② ③ ④ ⑤ ⑥ ⑦ ⑧ ⑨ ⑩
Mental Clarity	① ② ③ ④ ⑤ ⑥ ⑦ ⑧ ⑨ ⑩

PAIN & SYMPTOM DETAILS

	am	pm	front	back	other
	☐	☐			☐ Nausea
	☐	☐			☐ Diarrhea
	☐	☐			☐ Vomiting
	☐	☐			☐ Sore throat
	☐	☐			☐ Congestion
	☐	☐			☐ Coughing
	☐	☐			☐ Chills
	☐	☐			☐ Fever

SLEEP

hours _____

quality ① ② ③ ④ ⑤

STRESS LEVELS

None	Low	Medium	High	Max	@$#%!

WEATHER

☐ Cold   ☐ Mild   ☐ Hot
☐ Dry   ☐ Humid   ☐ Wet

Allergen Levels: _____
BM Pressure: _____

EXERCISE

☐ Heck yes, I worked out.
☐ I managed to exercise a bit.
☐ No, I haven't exercised at all.
☐ I did some stuff, and that counts.

DETAILS

FOOD / MEDICATION

Food / Drinks

Meds / Supplements	Time	Dose

☐ usual daily medication

Notes

I am grateful for...

M T W T F S S   DATE:

HOW ARE YOU *Feeling today?*

Amazing!	Meh
Great	Not good
Good	Terrible!

RATE YOUR PAIN LEVEL

① ② ③ ④ ⑤ ⑥ ⑦ ⑧ ⑨ ⑩

WHAT ABOUT YOUR...?

Mood	① ② ③ ④ ⑤ ⑥ ⑦ ⑧ ⑨ ⑩
Energy Levels	① ② ③ ④ ⑤ ⑥ ⑦ ⑧ ⑨ ⑩
Mental Clarity	① ② ③ ④ ⑤ ⑥ ⑦ ⑧ ⑨ ⑩

PAIN & SYMPTOM DETAILS

	am	pm	*front*	*back*	*other*
	☐	☐			☐ Nausea
	☐	☐			☐ Diarrhea
	☐	☐			☐ Vomiting
	☐	☐			☐ Sore throat
	☐	☐			☐ Congestion
	☐	☐			☐ Coughing
	☐	☐			☐ Chills
	☐	☐			☐ Fever

SLEEP

hours
_____

quality
① ② ③ ④ ⑤

STRESS LEVELS

None	Low	Medium	High	Max	@$#%!

WEATHER

☐ Cold   ☐ Mild   ☐ Hot
☐ Dry   ☐ Humid   ☐ Wet
Allergen Levels: _____
BM Pressure: _____

EXERCISE

☐ Heck yes, I worked out.
☐ I managed to exercise a bit.
☐ No, I haven't exercised at all.
☐ I did some stuff, and that counts.

DETAILS

FOOD / MEDICATION

Food / Drinks

Meds / Supplements	Time	Dose

☐ usual daily medication

Notes
_____

_____

I am grateful for...

HOW ARE YOU *Feeling today?*

😍 Amazing!	🙂 Meh
😁 Great	😠 Not good
😊 Good	😖 Terrible!

RATE YOUR PAIN LEVEL

① ② ③ ④ ⑤ ⑥ ⑦ ⑧ ⑨ ⑩

WHAT ABOUT YOUR...?

Mood	① ② ③ ④ ⑤ ⑥ ⑦ ⑧ ⑨ ⑩
Energy Levels	① ② ③ ④ ⑤ ⑥ ⑦ ⑧ ⑨ ⑩
Mental Clarity	① ② ③ ④ ⑤ ⑥ ⑦ ⑧ ⑨ ⑩

PAIN & SYMPTOM DETAILS

	am	pm	*front*	*back*	*other*
_____	☐	☐			☐ Nausea
_____	☐	☐			☐ Diarrhea
_____	☐	☐			☐ Vomiting
_____	☐	☐			☐ Sore throat
_____	☐	☐			☐ Congestion
_____	☐	☐			☐ Coughing
_____	☐	☐			☐ Chills
_____	☐	☐			☐ Fever

SLEEP

hours
_____

quality
① ② ③ ④ ⑤

STRESS LEVELS

None	Low	Medium	High	Max	@$#%!

WEATHER

☐ Cold   ☐ Mild   ☐ Hot
☐ Dry   ☐ Humid   ☐ Wet
Allergen Levels: _____
BM Pressure: _____

EXERCISE

☐ Heck yes, I worked out.
☐ I managed to exercise a bit.
☐ No, I haven't exercised at all.
☐ I did some stuff, and that counts.

DETAILS

FOOD / MEDICATION

Food / Drinks

Meds / Supplements	Time	Dose

☐ usual daily medication

Notes
_____
_____

I am grateful for...
_____

M T W T F S S

DATE:

HOW ARE YOU *Feeling today?*

😍 Amazing!	🙂 Meh
😁 Great	😠 Not good
🙂 Good	😣 Terrible!

RATE YOUR PAIN LEVEL

① ② ③ ④ ⑤ ⑥ ⑦ ⑧ ⑨ ⑩

WHAT ABOUT YOUR...?

Mood	① ② ③ ④ ⑤ ⑥ ⑦ ⑧ ⑨ ⑩
Energy Levels	① ② ③ ④ ⑤ ⑥ ⑦ ⑧ ⑨ ⑩
Mental Clarity	① ② ③ ④ ⑤ ⑥ ⑦ ⑧ ⑨ ⑩

PAIN & SYMPTOM DETAILS

	am	pm	*front*	*back*	*other*
_____	☐	☐			☐ Nausea
_____	☐	☐			☐ Diarrhea
_____	☐	☐			☐ Vomiting
_____	☐	☐			☐ Sore throat
_____	☐	☐			☐ Congestion
_____	☐	☐			☐ Coughing
_____	☐	☐			☐ Chills
_____	☐	☐			☐ Fever

SLEEP

hours
_____

quality
① ② ③ ④ ⑤

STRESS LEVELS

None	Low	Medium	High	Max	@$#%!

WEATHER

☐ Cold   ☐ Mild   ☐ Hot
☐ Dry   ☐ Humid   ☐ Wet
Allergen Levels: _____
BM Pressure: _____

EXERCISE

☐ Heck yes, I worked out.
☐ I managed to exercise a bit.
☐ No, I haven't exercised at all.
☐ I did some stuff, and that counts.

DETAILS

FOOD / MEDICATION

Food / Drinks

Meds / Supplements	Time	Dose

☐ usual daily medication

Notes
_____
_____

I am grateful for...

HOW ARE YOU *Feeling today?*

😍 Amazing!	🙂 Meh
😁 Great	😠 Not good
😊 Good	😖 Terrible!

RATE YOUR PAIN LEVEL

① ② ③ ④ ⑤ ⑥ ⑦ ⑧ ⑨ ⑩

WHAT ABOUT YOUR...?

Mood	① ② ③ ④ ⑤ ⑥ ⑦ ⑧ ⑨ ⑩
Energy Levels	① ② ③ ④ ⑤ ⑥ ⑦ ⑧ ⑨ ⑩
Mental Clarity	① ② ③ ④ ⑤ ⑥ ⑦ ⑧ ⑨ ⑩

PAIN & SYMPTOM DETAILS

	am	pm	*front*	*back*	*other*
_____	☐	☐			☐ Nausea
_____	☐	☐			☐ Diarrhea
_____	☐	☐			☐ Vomiting
_____	☐	☐			☐ Sore throat
_____	☐	☐			☐ Congestion
_____	☐	☐			☐ Coughing
_____	☐	☐			☐ Chills
_____	☐	☐			☐ Fever

SLEEP

hours _____

quality ① ② ③ ④ ⑤

STRESS LEVELS

None	Low	Medium	High	Max	@$#%!

WEATHER

☐ Cold ☐ Mild ☐ Hot
☐ Dry   ☐ Humid ☐ Wet
Allergen Levels: _____
BM Pressure: _____

EXERCISE

☐ Heck yes, I worked out.
☐ I managed to exercise a bit.
☐ No, I haven't exercised at all.
☐ I did some stuff, and that counts.

DETAILS

FOOD / MEDICATION

Food / Drinks

Meds / Supplements	Time	Dose

☐ usual daily medication

Notes
_____
_____

I am grateful for...
_____

HOW ARE YOU *Feeling today?*

😍 Amazing!	🙂 Meh
😁 Great	😠 Not good
🙂 Good	😖 Terrible!

RATE YOUR PAIN LEVEL

① ② ③ ④ ⑤ ⑥ ⑦ ⑧ ⑨ ⑩

WHAT ABOUT YOUR...?

Mood	① ② ③ ④ ⑤ ⑥ ⑦ ⑧ ⑨ ⑩
Energy Levels	① ② ③ ④ ⑤ ⑥ ⑦ ⑧ ⑨ ⑩
Mental Clarity	① ② ③ ④ ⑤ ⑥ ⑦ ⑧ ⑨ ⑩

PAIN & SYMPTOM DETAILS

	am	pm	*front*	*back*	*other*
_____	☐	☐			☐ Nausea
_____	☐	☐			☐ Diarrhea
_____	☐	☐			☐ Vomiting
_____	☐	☐			☐ Sore throat
_____	☐	☐			☐ Congestion
_____	☐	☐			☐ Coughing
_____	☐	☐			☐ Chills
_____	☐	☐			☐ Fever

SLEEP

hours
_____

quality
① ② ③ ④ ⑤

STRESS LEVELS

None	Low	Medium	High	Max	@$#%!

WEATHER

☐ Cold ☐ Mild ☐ Hot
☐ Dry ☐ Humid ☐ Wet

Allergen Levels: _____
BM Pressure: _____

EXERCISE

☐ Heck yes, I worked out.
☐ I managed to exercise a bit.
☐ No, I haven't exercised at all.
☐ I did some stuff, and that counts.

DETAILS

FOOD / MEDICATION

Food / Drinks

Meds / Supplements	Time	Dose

☐ usual daily medication

Notes

_____

I am grateful for...

M T W T F S S

DATE:

HOW ARE YOU Feeling today?

😍 Amazing!	🙂 Meh
😁 Great	😣 Not good
😊 Good	😖 Terrible!

RATE YOUR PAIN LEVEL

① ② ③ ④ ⑤ ⑥ ⑦ ⑧ ⑨ ⑩

WHAT ABOUT YOUR...?

Mood	① ② ③ ④ ⑤ ⑥ ⑦ ⑧ ⑨ ⑩
Energy Levels	① ② ③ ④ ⑤ ⑥ ⑦ ⑧ ⑨ ⑩
Mental Clarity	① ② ③ ④ ⑤ ⑥ ⑦ ⑧ ⑨ ⑩

PAIN & SYMPTOM DETAILS

	am	pm	front	back	other
	☐	☐			☐ Nausea
	☐	☐			☐ Diarrhea
	☐	☐			☐ Vomiting
	☐	☐			☐ Sore throat
	☐	☐			☐ Congestion
	☐	☐			☐ Coughing
	☐	☐			☐ Chills
	☐	☐			☐ Fever

SLEEP

hours
_____

quality
① ② ③ ④ ⑤

STRESS LEVELS

None	Low	Medium	High	Max	@$#%!

WEATHER

☐ Cold ☐ Mild ☐ Hot
☐ Dry ☐ Humid ☐ Wet

Allergen Levels: _____
BM Pressure: _____

EXERCISE

☐ Heck yes, I worked out.
☐ I managed to exercise a bit.
☐ No, I haven't exercised at all.
☐ I did some stuff, and that counts.

DETAILS

FOOD / MEDICATION

Food / Drinks

Meds / Supplements	Time	Dose

☐ usual daily medication

Notes
_____
_____

I am grateful for...

HOW ARE YOU *Feeling today?*

Amazing!	Meh
Great	Not good
Good	Terrible!

RATE YOUR PAIN LEVEL

① ② ③ ④ ⑤ ⑥ ⑦ ⑧ ⑨ ⑩

WHAT ABOUT YOUR...?

Mood	① ② ③ ④ ⑤ ⑥ ⑦ ⑧ ⑨ ⑩
Energy Levels	① ② ③ ④ ⑤ ⑥ ⑦ ⑧ ⑨ ⑩
Mental Clarity	① ② ③ ④ ⑤ ⑥ ⑦ ⑧ ⑨ ⑩

PAIN & SYMPTOM DETAILS

	am	pm	*front*	*back*	*other*
	☐	☐			☐ Nausea
	☐	☐			☐ Diarrhea
	☐	☐			☐ Vomiting
	☐	☐			☐ Sore throat
	☐	☐			☐ Congestion
	☐	☐			☐ Coughing
	☐	☐			☐ Chills
	☐	☐			☐ Fever

SLEEP

hours _____

quality ① ② ③ ④ ⑤

STRESS LEVELS

None	Low	Medium	High	Max	@$#%!

WEATHER

☐ Cold   ☐ Mild   ☐ Hot
☐ Dry   ☐ Humid ☐ Wet

Allergen Levels: _____
BM Pressure: _____

EXERCISE

☐ Heck yes, I worked out.
☐ I managed to exercise a bit.
☐ No, I haven't exercised at all.
☐ I did some stuff, and that counts.

DETAILS

FOOD / MEDICATION

Food / Drinks

Meds / Supplements	Time	Dose

☐ usual daily medication

Notes

_____

_____

I am grateful for...

HOW ARE YOU *Feeling today?*

Amazing!	Meh
Great	Not good
Good	Terrible!

RATE YOUR PAIN LEVEL

① ② ③ ④ ⑤ ⑥ ⑦ ⑧ ⑨ ⑩

WHAT ABOUT YOUR...?

Mood	① ② ③ ④ ⑤ ⑥ ⑦ ⑧ ⑨ ⑩
Energy Levels	① ② ③ ④ ⑤ ⑥ ⑦ ⑧ ⑨ ⑩
Mental Clarity	① ② ③ ④ ⑤ ⑥ ⑦ ⑧ ⑨ ⑩

PAIN & SYMPTOM DETAILS

	am	pm	*front*	*back*	*other*
	☐	☐			☐ Nausea
	☐	☐			☐ Diarrhea
	☐	☐			☐ Vomiting
	☐	☐			☐ Sore throat
	☐	☐			☐ Congestion
	☐	☐			☐ Coughing
	☐	☐			☐ Chills
	☐	☐			☐ Fever

SLEEP

hours _____   *quality* ① ② ③ ④ ⑤

STRESS LEVELS

None	Low	Medium	High	Max	@$#%!

WEATHER

☐ Cold   ☐ Mild   ☐ Hot
☐ Dry   ☐ Humid   ☐ Wet
Allergen Levels: _____
BM Pressure: _____

EXERCISE

☐ Heck yes, I worked out.
☐ I managed to exercise a bit.
☐ No, I haven't exercised at all.
☐ I did some stuff, and that counts.

DETAILS

FOOD / MEDICATION

Food / Drinks

Meds / Supplements	Time	Dose

☐ usual daily medication

Notes

I am grateful for...

HOW ARE YOU *Feeling today?*

😍 Amazing!	🙂 Meh
😁 Great	😠 Not good
🙂 Good	😣 Terrible!

RATE YOUR PAIN LEVEL

(1) (2) (3) (4) (5) (6) (7) (8) (9) (10)

WHAT ABOUT YOUR...?

Mood	(1) (2) (3) (4) (5) (6) (7) (8) (9) (10)
Energy Levels	(1) (2) (3) (4) (5) (6) (7) (8) (9) (10)
Mental Clarity	(1) (2) (3) (4) (5) (6) (7) (8) (9) (10)

PAIN & SYMPTOM DETAILS

	am	pm	*front*	*back*	*other*
_____	☐	☐			☐ Nausea
_____	☐	☐			☐ Diarrhea
_____	☐	☐			☐ Vomiting
_____	☐	☐			☐ Sore throat
_____	☐	☐			☐ Congestion
_____	☐	☐			☐ Coughing
_____	☐	☐			☐ Chills
_____	☐	☐			☐ Fever

SLEEP

hours
_____

quality
(1) (2) (3) (4) (5)

STRESS LEVELS

None	Low	Medium	High	Max	@$#%!

WEATHER

☐ Cold   ☐ Mild   ☐ Hot
☐ Dry   ☐ Humid   ☐ Wet
Allergen Levels: _____
BM Pressure: _____

EXERCISE

☐ Heck yes, I worked out.
☐ I managed to exercise a bit.
☐ No, I haven't exercised at all.
☐ I did some stuff, and that counts.

DETAILS

FOOD / MEDICATION

Food / Drinks

Meds / Supplements	Time	Dose

☐ usual daily medication

Notes
_____
_____

I am grateful for...

HOW ARE YOU *Feeling today?*

Amazing!	Meh
Great	Not good
Good	Terrible!

RATE YOUR PAIN LEVEL

(1) (2) (3) (4) (5) (6) (7) (8) (9) (10)

WHAT ABOUT YOUR...?

Mood	(1) (2) (3) (4) (5) (6) (7) (8) (9) (10)
Energy Levels	(1) (2) (3) (4) (5) (6) (7) (8) (9) (10)
Mental Clarity	(1) (2) (3) (4) (5) (6) (7) (8) (9) (10)

PAIN & SYMPTOM DETAILS

	am	pm	*front*	*back*	*other*
_____	☐	☐			☐ Nausea
_____	☐	☐			☐ Diarrhea
_____	☐	☐			☐ Vomiting
_____	☐	☐			☐ Sore throat
_____	☐	☐			☐ Congestion
_____	☐	☐			☐ Coughing
_____	☐	☐			☐ Chills
_____	☐	☐			☐ Fever

SLEEP

hours
_____

quality
(1) (2) (3) (4) (5)

STRESS LEVELS

None	Low	Medium	High	Max	@$#%!

WEATHER

☐ Cold ☐ Mild ☐ Hot
☐ Dry ☐ Humid ☐ Wet
Allergen Levels: _____
BM Pressure: _____

EXERCISE

☐ Heck yes, I worked out.
☐ I managed to exercise a bit.
☐ No, I haven't exercised at all.
☐ I did some stuff, and that counts.

DETAILS

FOOD / MEDICATION

Food / Drinks

Meds / Supplements	Time	Dose
☐ usual daily medication		

Notes
_____

I am grateful for...

M T W T F S S DATE:

HOW ARE YOU *Feeling today?*

Amazing!	Meh
Great	Not good
Good	Terrible!

RATE YOUR PAIN LEVEL

(1) (2) (3) (4) (5) (6) (7) (8) (9) (10)

WHAT ABOUT YOUR...?

Mood	(1) (2) (3) (4) (5) (6) (7) (8) (9) (10)
Energy Levels	(1) (2) (3) (4) (5) (6) (7) (8) (9) (10)
Mental Clarity	(1) (2) (3) (4) (5) (6) (7) (8) (9) (10)

PAIN & SYMPTOM DETAILS

	am	pm	*front*	*back*	*other*
_____	☐	☐			☐ Nausea
_____	☐	☐			☐ Diarrhea
_____	☐	☐			☐ Vomiting
_____	☐	☐			☐ Sore throat
_____	☐	☐			☐ Congestion
_____	☐	☐			☐ Coughing
_____	☐	☐			☐ Chills
_____	☐	☐			☐ Fever

SLEEP

hours
_____

quality
(1) (2) (3) (4) (5)

STRESS LEVELS

None	Low	Medium	High	Max	@$#%!

WEATHER

☐ Cold   ☐ Mild   ☐ Hot
☐ Dry   ☐ Humid   ☐ Wet

Allergen Levels: _____
BM Pressure: _____

EXERCISE

☐ Heck yes, I worked out.
☐ I managed to exercise a bit.
☐ No, I haven't exercised at all.
☐ I did some stuff, and that counts.

DETAILS

FOOD / MEDICATION

Food / Drinks

Meds / Supplements	Time	Dose

☐ usual daily medication

Notes
_____
_____

I am grateful for...

HOW ARE YOU *Feeling today?*

😍 Amazing!	🙂 Meh
😁 Great	😠 Not good
😊 Good	😖 Terrible!

RATE YOUR PAIN LEVEL

①②③④⑤⑥⑦⑧⑨⑩

WHAT ABOUT YOUR...?

Mood	①②③④⑤⑥⑦⑧⑨⑩
Energy Levels	①②③④⑤⑥⑦⑧⑨⑩
Mental Clarity	①②③④⑤⑥⑦⑧⑨⑩

PAIN & SYMPTOM DETAILS

	am	pm	front	back	other
_____	☐	☐			☐ Nausea
_____	☐	☐			☐ Diarrhea
_____	☐	☐			☐ Vomiting
_____	☐	☐			☐ Sore throat
_____	☐	☐			☐ Congestion
_____	☐	☐			☐ Coughing
_____	☐	☐			☐ Chills
_____	☐	☐			☐ Fever

SLEEP

hours
_____

quality
① ② ③ ④ ⑤

STRESS LEVELS

None	Low	Medium	High	Max	@$#%!

WEATHER

☐ Cold   ☐ Mild   ☐ Hot
☐ Dry   ☐ Humid   ☐ Wet

Allergen Levels: _____
BM Pressure: _____

EXERCISE

☐ Heck yes, I worked out.
☐ I managed to exercise a bit.
☐ No, I haven't exercised at all.
☐ I did some stuff, and that counts.

DETAILS

FOOD / MEDICATION

Food / Drinks

Meds / Supplements	Time	Dose

☐ usual daily medication

Notes
_____

I am grateful for...
_____

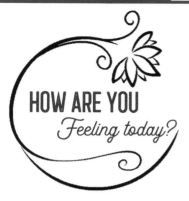

HOW ARE YOU *Feeling today?*

☺ Amazing!	☺ Meh
😁 Great	😠 Not good
🙂 Good	😖 Terrible!

RATE YOUR PAIN LEVEL

① ② ③ ④ ⑤ ⑥ ⑦ ⑧ ⑨ ⑩

WHAT ABOUT YOUR...?

Mood	① ② ③ ④ ⑤ ⑥ ⑦ ⑧ ⑨ ⑩
Energy Levels	① ② ③ ④ ⑤ ⑥ ⑦ ⑧ ⑨ ⑩
Mental Clarity	① ② ③ ④ ⑤ ⑥ ⑦ ⑧ ⑨ ⑩

PAIN & SYMPTOM DETAILS

	am	pm	*front*	*back*	*other*
	☐	☐			☐ Nausea
	☐	☐			☐ Diarrhea
	☐	☐			☐ Vomiting
	☐	☐			☐ Sore throat
	☐	☐			☐ Congestion
	☐	☐			☐ Coughing
	☐	☐			☐ Chills
	☐	☐			☐ Fever

SLEEP

hours
_____

quality
① ② ③ ④ ⑤

STRESS LEVELS

None	Low	Medium	High	Max	@$#%!

WEATHER

☐ Cold   ☐ Mild   ☐ Hot
☐ Dry   ☐ Humid   ☐ Wet
Allergen Levels: _____
BM Pressure: _____

EXERCISE

☐ Heck yes, I worked out.
☐ I managed to exercise a bit.
☐ No, I haven't exercised at all.
☐ I did some stuff, and that counts.

DETAILS

FOOD / MEDICATION

Food / Drinks

Meds / Supplements	Time	Dose

☐ usual daily medication

Notes
_____

I am grateful for...
_____

M T W T F S S

DATE:

HOW ARE YOU Feeling today?

Amazing!	Meh
Great	Not good
Good	Terrible!

RATE YOUR PAIN LEVEL

① ② ③ ④ ⑤ ⑥ ⑦ ⑧ ⑨ ⑩

WHAT ABOUT YOUR...?

Mood	① ② ③ ④ ⑤ ⑥ ⑦ ⑧ ⑨ ⑩
Energy Levels	① ② ③ ④ ⑤ ⑥ ⑦ ⑧ ⑨ ⑩
Mental Clarity	① ② ③ ④ ⑤ ⑥ ⑦ ⑧ ⑨ ⑩

PAIN & SYMPTOM DETAILS

	am	pm	*front*	*back*	*other*
	☐	☐			☐ Nausea
	☐	☐			☐ Diarrhea
	☐	☐			☐ Vomiting
	☐	☐			☐ Sore throat
	☐	☐			☐ Congestion
	☐	☐			☐ Coughing
	☐	☐			☐ Chills
	☐	☐			☐ Fever

SLEEP

hours
_____

quality
① ② ③ ④ ⑤

STRESS LEVELS

None	Low	Medium	High	Max	@$#%!

WEATHER

☐ Cold   ☐ Mild   ☐ Hot
☐ Dry   ☐ Humid   ☐ Wet

Allergen Levels: _____
BM Pressure: _____

EXERCISE

☐ Heck yes, I worked out.
☐ I managed to exercise a bit.
☐ No, I haven't exercised at all.
☐ I did some stuff, and that counts.

DETAILS

FOOD / MEDICATION

Food / Drinks

Meds / Supplements	Time	Dose

☐ usual daily medication

Notes
_____
_____

I am grateful for...
_____

M T W T F S S   DATE:

HOW ARE YOU Feeling today?

Amazing!	Meh
Great	Not good
Good	Terrible!

RATE YOUR PAIN LEVEL

① ② ③ ④ ⑤ ⑥ ⑦ ⑧ ⑨ ⑩

WHAT ABOUT YOUR...?

Mood	① ② ③ ④ ⑤ ⑥ ⑦ ⑧ ⑨ ⑩
Energy Levels	① ② ③ ④ ⑤ ⑥ ⑦ ⑧ ⑨ ⑩
Mental Clarity	① ② ③ ④ ⑤ ⑥ ⑦ ⑧ ⑨ ⑩

PAIN & SYMPTOM DETAILS

	am	pm	front	back	other
	☐	☐			☐ Nausea
	☐	☐			☐ Diarrhea
	☐	☐			☐ Vomiting
	☐	☐			☐ Sore throat
	☐	☐			☐ Congestion
	☐	☐			☐ Coughing
	☐	☐			☐ Chills
	☐	☐			☐ Fever

SLEEP

hours   quality
_____   ① ② ③ ④ ⑤

STRESS LEVELS

| None | Low | Medium | High | Max | @$#%! |

WEATHER

☐ Cold   ☐ Mild   ☐ Hot
☐ Dry   ☐ Humid   ☐ Wet
Allergen Levels: _____
BM Pressure: _____

EXERCISE

☐ Heck yes, I worked out.
☐ I managed to exercise a bit.
☐ No, I haven't exercised at all.
☐ I did some stuff, and that counts.

DETAILS

FOOD / MEDICATION

Food / Drinks

Meds / Supplements	Time	Dose

☐ usual daily medication

Notes
_____
_____

I am grateful for...

HOW ARE YOU *Feeling today?*

Amazing!	Meh
Great	Not good
Good	Terrible!

RATE YOUR PAIN LEVEL

① ② ③ ④ ⑤ ⑥ ⑦ ⑧ ⑨ ⑩

WHAT ABOUT YOUR...?

Mood	① ② ③ ④ ⑤ ⑥ ⑦ ⑧ ⑨ ⑩	
Energy Levels	① ② ③ ④ ⑤ ⑥ ⑦ ⑧ ⑨ ⑩	
Mental Clarity	① ② ③ ④ ⑤ ⑥ ⑦ ⑧ ⑨ ⑩	

PAIN & SYMPTOM DETAILS

	am	pm	*front*	*back*	*other*
_____	☐	☐			☐ Nausea
_____	☐	☐			☐ Diarrhea
_____	☐	☐			☐ Vomiting
_____	☐	☐			☐ Sore throat
_____	☐	☐			☐ Congestion
_____	☐	☐			☐ Coughing
_____	☐	☐			☐ Chills
_____	☐	☐			☐ Fever

SLEEP

hours _____

quality ① ② ③ ④ ⑤

STRESS LEVELS

None	Low	Medium	High	Max	@$#%!

WEATHER

☐ Cold ☐ Mild ☐ Hot
☐ Dry ☐ Humid ☐ Wet

Allergen Levels: _____
BM Pressure: _____

EXERCISE

☐ Heck yes, I worked out.
☐ I managed to exercise a bit.
☐ No, I haven't exercised at all.
☐ I did some stuff, and that counts.

DETAILS

FOOD / MEDICATION

Food / Drinks	Meds / Supplements	Time	Dose

☐ usual daily medication

Notes
_____
_____

I am grateful for...
_____

HOW ARE YOU Feeling today?

😍 Amazing!	🙂 Meh
😁 Great	😠 Not good
😊 Good	😖 Terrible!

RATE YOUR PAIN LEVEL

① ② ③ ④ ⑤ ⑥ ⑦ ⑧ ⑨ ⑩

WHAT ABOUT YOUR...?

Mood	① ② ③ ④ ⑤ ⑥ ⑦ ⑧ ⑨ ⑩
Energy Levels	① ② ③ ④ ⑤ ⑥ ⑦ ⑧ ⑨ ⑩
Mental Clarity	① ② ③ ④ ⑤ ⑥ ⑦ ⑧ ⑨ ⑩

PAIN & SYMPTOM DETAILS

	am	pm	front	back	other
	☐	☐			☐ Nausea
	☐	☐			☐ Diarrhea
	☐	☐			☐ Vomiting
	☐	☐			☐ Sore throat
	☐	☐			☐ Congestion
	☐	☐			☐ Coughing
	☐	☐			☐ Chills
	☐	☐			☐ Fever

SLEEP

hours
_____

quality
① ② ③ ④ ⑤

STRESS LEVELS

None	Low	Medium	High	Max	@$#%!

WEATHER

☐ Cold   ☐ Mild   ☐ Hot
☐ Dry   ☐ Humid   ☐ Wet
Allergen Levels: _____
BM Pressure: _____

EXERCISE

☐ Heck yes, I worked out.
☐ I managed to exercise a bit.
☐ No, I haven't exercised at all.
☐ I did some stuff, and that counts.

DETAILS

FOOD / MEDICATION

Food / Drinks

Meds / Supplements	Time	Dose

☐ usual daily medication

Notes
_____
_____

I am grateful for...
_____

HOW ARE YOU Feeling today?

Amazing!	Meh
Great	Not good
Good	Terrible!

RATE YOUR PAIN LEVEL

① ② ③ ④ ⑤ ⑥ ⑦ ⑧ ⑨ ⑩

WHAT ABOUT YOUR...?

Mood	① ② ③ ④ ⑤ ⑥ ⑦ ⑧ ⑨ ⑩
Energy Levels	① ② ③ ④ ⑤ ⑥ ⑦ ⑧ ⑨ ⑩
Mental Clarity	① ② ③ ④ ⑤ ⑥ ⑦ ⑧ ⑨ ⑩

PAIN & SYMPTOM DETAILS

	am	pm	front	back	other
	☐	☐			☐ Nausea
	☐	☐			☐ Diarrhea
	☐	☐			☐ Vomiting
	☐	☐			☐ Sore throat
	☐	☐			☐ Congestion
	☐	☐			☐ Coughing
	☐	☐			☐ Chills
	☐	☐			☐ Fever

SLEEP

hours _____   *quality* ① ② ③ ④ ⑤

STRESS LEVELS

None	Low	Medium	High	Max	@$#%!

WEATHER

☐ Cold   ☐ Mild   ☐ Hot
☐ Dry   ☐ Humid   ☐ Wet
Allergen Levels: _____
BM Pressure: _____

EXERCISE

☐ Heck yes, I worked out.
☐ I managed to exercise a bit.
☐ No, I haven't exercised at all.
☐ I did some stuff, and that counts.

DETAILS

FOOD / MEDICATION

Food / Drinks	Meds / Supplements	Time	Dose

☐ usual daily medication

Notes

I am grateful for...

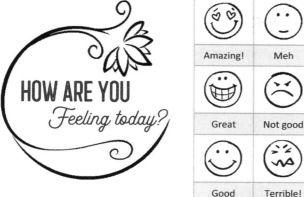

HOW ARE YOU *Feeling today?*

☺ Amazing!	☺ Meh
😁 Great	😠 Not good
🙂 Good	😝 Terrible!

RATE YOUR PAIN LEVEL

① ② ③ ④ ⑤ ⑥ ⑦ ⑧ ⑨ ⑩

WHAT ABOUT YOUR...?

Mood	① ② ③ ④ ⑤ ⑥ ⑦ ⑧ ⑨ ⑩
Energy Levels	① ② ③ ④ ⑤ ⑥ ⑦ ⑧ ⑨ ⑩
Mental Clarity	① ② ③ ④ ⑤ ⑥ ⑦ ⑧ ⑨ ⑩

PAIN & SYMPTOM DETAILS

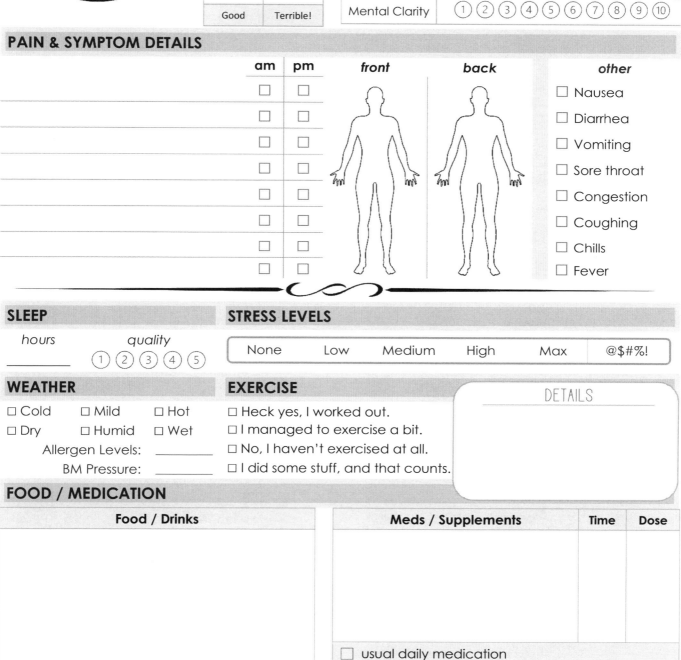

	am	pm		*front*	*back*		*other*
_____	☐	☐					☐ Nausea
_____	☐	☐					☐ Diarrhea
_____	☐	☐					☐ Vomiting
_____	☐	☐					☐ Sore throat
_____	☐	☐					☐ Congestion
_____	☐	☐					☐ Coughing
_____	☐	☐					☐ Chills
_____	☐	☐					☐ Fever

SLEEP

hours _____

quality ① ② ③ ④ ⑤

STRESS LEVELS

None	Low	Medium	High	Max	@$#%!

WEATHER

☐ Cold   ☐ Mild   ☐ Hot
☐ Dry   ☐ Humid   ☐ Wet

Allergen Levels: _____
BM Pressure: _____

EXERCISE

☐ Heck yes, I worked out.
☐ I managed to exercise a bit.
☐ No, I haven't exercised at all.
☐ I did some stuff, and that counts.

DETAILS

FOOD / MEDICATION

Food / Drinks

Meds / Supplements	Time	Dose

☐ usual daily medication

Notes
_____

I am grateful for...

HOW ARE YOU *Feeling today?*

Amazing!	Meh
Great	Not good
Good	Terrible!

RATE YOUR PAIN LEVEL

① ② ③ ④ ⑤ ⑥ ⑦ ⑧ ⑨ ⑩

WHAT ABOUT YOUR...?

Mood	① ② ③ ④ ⑤ ⑥ ⑦ ⑧ ⑨ ⑩
Energy Levels	① ② ③ ④ ⑤ ⑥ ⑦ ⑧ ⑨ ⑩
Mental Clarity	① ② ③ ④ ⑤ ⑥ ⑦ ⑧ ⑨ ⑩

PAIN & SYMPTOM DETAILS

	am	pm	*front*	*back*	other
	☐	☐			☐ Nausea
	☐	☐			☐ Diarrhea
	☐	☐			☐ Vomiting
	☐	☐			☐ Sore throat
	☐	☐			☐ Congestion
	☐	☐			☐ Coughing
	☐	☐			☐ Chills
	☐	☐			☐ Fever

SLEEP

hours _____

quality ① ② ③ ④ ⑤

STRESS LEVELS

None	Low	Medium	High	Max	@$#%!

WEATHER

☐ Cold ☐ Mild ☐ Hot
☐ Dry ☐ Humid ☐ Wet

Allergen Levels: _____
BM Pressure: _____

EXERCISE

☐ Heck yes, I worked out.
☐ I managed to exercise a bit.
☐ No, I haven't exercised at all.
☐ I did some stuff, and that counts.

DETAILS

FOOD / MEDICATION

Food / Drinks	Meds / Supplements	Time	Dose

☐ usual daily medication

Notes

I am grateful for...

HOW ARE YOU *Feeling today?*

😍 Amazing!	🙂 Meh
😁 Great	😠 Not good
🙂 Good	😖 Terrible!

RATE YOUR PAIN LEVEL

① ② ③ ④ ⑤ ⑥ ⑦ ⑧ ⑨ ⑩

WHAT ABOUT YOUR...?

Mood	① ② ③ ④ ⑤ ⑥ ⑦ ⑧ ⑨ ⑩
Energy Levels	① ② ③ ④ ⑤ ⑥ ⑦ ⑧ ⑨ ⑩
Mental Clarity	① ② ③ ④ ⑤ ⑥ ⑦ ⑧ ⑨ ⑩

PAIN & SYMPTOM DETAILS

	am	pm	*front*	*back*	*other*
_____	☐	☐			☐ Nausea
_____	☐	☐			☐ Diarrhea
_____	☐	☐			☐ Vomiting
_____	☐	☐			☐ Sore throat
_____	☐	☐			☐ Congestion
_____	☐	☐			☐ Coughing
_____	☐	☐			☐ Chills
_____	☐	☐			☐ Fever

SLEEP

hours
_____

quality
① ② ③ ④ ⑤

STRESS LEVELS

None	Low	Medium	High	Max	@$#%!

WEATHER

☐ Cold   ☐ Mild   ☐ Hot
☐ Dry   ☐ Humid   ☐ Wet
Allergen Levels: _____
BM Pressure: _____

EXERCISE

☐ Heck yes, I worked out.
☐ I managed to exercise a bit.
☐ No, I haven't exercised at all.
☐ I did some stuff, and that counts.

DETAILS

FOOD / MEDICATION

Food / Drinks

Meds / Supplements	Time	Dose

☐ usual daily medication

Notes

_____

_____

I am grateful for...

M T W T F S S   DATE:

HOW ARE YOU *Feeling today?*

😍 Amazing!	🙂 Meh
😁 Great	😠 Not good
😊 Good	😤 Terrible!

RATE YOUR PAIN LEVEL

① ② ③ ④ ⑤ ⑥ ⑦ ⑧ ⑨ ⑩

WHAT ABOUT YOUR...?

Mood	① ② ③ ④ ⑤ ⑥ ⑦ ⑧ ⑨ ⑩
Energy Levels	① ② ③ ④ ⑤ ⑥ ⑦ ⑧ ⑨ ⑩
Mental Clarity	① ② ③ ④ ⑤ ⑥ ⑦ ⑧ ⑨ ⑩

PAIN & SYMPTOM DETAILS

	am	pm	front	back	other
	☐	☐			☐ Nausea
	☐	☐			☐ Diarrhea
	☐	☐			☐ Vomiting
	☐	☐			☐ Sore throat
	☐	☐			☐ Congestion
	☐	☐			☐ Coughing
	☐	☐			☐ Chills
	☐	☐			☐ Fever

SLEEP

hours _____   *quality* ① ② ③ ④ ⑤

STRESS LEVELS

None	Low	Medium	High	Max	@$#%!

WEATHER

☐ Cold   ☐ Mild   ☐ Hot
☐ Dry   ☐ Humid   ☐ Wet
Allergen Levels: _____
BM Pressure: _____

EXERCISE

☐ Heck yes, I worked out.
☐ I managed to exercise a bit.
☐ No, I haven't exercised at all.
☐ I did some stuff, and that counts.

DETAILS

FOOD / MEDICATION

Food / Drinks	Meds / Supplements	Time	Dose

☐ usual daily medication

Notes

I am grateful for...

HOW ARE YOU *Feeling today?*

😍 Amazing!	🙂 Meh
😁 Great	😠 Not good
😊 Good	😖 Terrible!

RATE YOUR PAIN LEVEL

① ② ③ ④ ⑤ ⑥ ⑦ ⑧ ⑨ ⑩

WHAT ABOUT YOUR...?

Mood	① ② ③ ④ ⑤ ⑥ ⑦ ⑧ ⑨ ⑩
Energy Levels	① ② ③ ④ ⑤ ⑥ ⑦ ⑧ ⑨ ⑩
Mental Clarity	① ② ③ ④ ⑤ ⑥ ⑦ ⑧ ⑨ ⑩

PAIN & SYMPTOM DETAILS

	am	pm
	☐	☐
	☐	☐
	☐	☐
	☐	☐
	☐	☐
	☐	☐
	☐	☐
	☐	☐

front   *back*

other

- ☐ Nausea
- ☐ Diarrhea
- ☐ Vomiting
- ☐ Sore throat
- ☐ Congestion
- ☐ Coughing
- ☐ Chills
- ☐ Fever

SLEEP

hours _____

quality ① ② ③ ④ ⑤

STRESS LEVELS

None	Low	Medium	High	Max	@$#%!

WEATHER

- ☐ Cold
- ☐ Dry
- ☐ Mild
- ☐ Humid
- ☐ Hot
- ☐ Wet

Allergen Levels: _____

BM Pressure: _____

EXERCISE

- ☐ Heck yes, I worked out.
- ☐ I managed to exercise a bit.
- ☐ No, I haven't exercised at all.
- ☐ I did some stuff, and that counts.

DETAILS

FOOD / MEDICATION

Food / Drinks

Meds / Supplements	Time	Dose

☐ usual daily medication

Notes

I am grateful for...

M T W T F S S | DATE:

HOW ARE YOU Feeling today?

😍 Amazing!	🙂 Meh
😁 Great	😠 Not good
🙂 Good	😖 Terrible!

RATE YOUR PAIN LEVEL

① ② ③ ④ ⑤ ⑥ ⑦ ⑧ ⑨ ⑩

WHAT ABOUT YOUR...?

Mood	① ② ③ ④ ⑤ ⑥ ⑦ ⑧ ⑨ ⑩
Energy Levels	① ② ③ ④ ⑤ ⑥ ⑦ ⑧ ⑨ ⑩
Mental Clarity	① ② ③ ④ ⑤ ⑥ ⑦ ⑧ ⑨ ⑩

PAIN & SYMPTOM DETAILS

	am	pm	front	back	other
_____	☐	☐			☐ Nausea
_____	☐	☐			☐ Diarrhea
_____	☐	☐			☐ Vomiting
_____	☐	☐			☐ Sore throat
_____	☐	☐			☐ Congestion
_____	☐	☐			☐ Coughing
_____	☐	☐			☐ Chills
_____	☐	☐			☐ Fever

SLEEP

hours _____   quality ① ② ③ ④ ⑤

STRESS LEVELS

None	Low	Medium	High	Max	@$#%!

WEATHER

☐ Cold ☐ Mild ☐ Hot
☐ Dry ☐ Humid ☐ Wet
Allergen Levels: _____
BM Pressure: _____

EXERCISE

☐ Heck yes, I worked out.
☐ I managed to exercise a bit.
☐ No, I haven't exercised at all.
☐ I did some stuff, and that counts.

DETAILS

FOOD / MEDICATION

Food / Drinks	Meds / Supplements	Time	Dose

☐ usual daily medication

Notes
_____

I am grateful for...

HOW ARE YOU Feeling today?

Amazing!	Meh
Great	Not good
Good	Terrible!

RATE YOUR PAIN LEVEL
① ② ③ ④ ⑤ ⑥ ⑦ ⑧ ⑨ ⑩

WHAT ABOUT YOUR...?

Mood	① ② ③ ④ ⑤ ⑥ ⑦ ⑧ ⑨ ⑩	
Energy Levels	① ② ③ ④ ⑤ ⑥ ⑦ ⑧ ⑨ ⑩	
Mental Clarity	① ② ③ ④ ⑤ ⑥ ⑦ ⑧ ⑨ ⑩	

PAIN & SYMPTOM DETAILS

	am	pm	front	back	other
	☐	☐			☐ Nausea
	☐	☐			☐ Diarrhea
	☐	☐			☐ Vomiting
	☐	☐			☐ Sore throat
	☐	☐			☐ Congestion
	☐	☐			☐ Coughing
	☐	☐			☐ Chills
	☐	☐			☐ Fever

SLEEP

hours _____

quality ① ② ③ ④ ⑤

STRESS LEVELS

None	Low	Medium	High	Max	@$#%!

WEATHER

☐ Cold   ☐ Mild   ☐ Hot
☐ Dry   ☐ Humid   ☐ Wet
Allergen Levels: _____
BM Pressure: _____

EXERCISE

☐ Heck yes, I worked out.
☐ I managed to exercise a bit.
☐ No, I haven't exercised at all.
☐ I did some stuff, and that counts.

DETAILS

FOOD / MEDICATION

Food / Drinks

Meds / Supplements	Time	Dose

☐ usual daily medication

Notes

I am grateful for...

HOW ARE YOU *Feeling today?*

Amazing!	Meh
Great	Not good
Good	Terrible!

RATE YOUR PAIN LEVEL

(1) (2) (3) (4) (5) (6) (7) (8) (9) (10)

WHAT ABOUT YOUR...?

Mood	(1) (2) (3) (4) (5) (6) (7) (8) (9) (10)
Energy Levels	(1) (2) (3) (4) (5) (6) (7) (8) (9) (10)
Mental Clarity	(1) (2) (3) (4) (5) (6) (7) (8) (9) (10)

PAIN & SYMPTOM DETAILS

	am	pm	*front*	*back*	*other*
	☐	☐			☐ Nausea
	☐	☐			☐ Diarrhea
	☐	☐			☐ Vomiting
	☐	☐			☐ Sore throat
	☐	☐			☐ Congestion
	☐	☐			☐ Coughing
	☐	☐			☐ Chills
	☐	☐			☐ Fever

SLEEP

hours _____   *quality* (1) (2) (3) (4) (5)

STRESS LEVELS

None	Low	Medium	High	Max	@$#%!

WEATHER

☐ Cold ☐ Mild ☐ Hot
☐ Dry ☐ Humid ☐ Wet
Allergen Levels: _____
BM Pressure: _____

EXERCISE

☐ Heck yes, I worked out.
☐ I managed to exercise a bit.
☐ No, I haven't exercised at all.
☐ I did some stuff, and that counts.

DETAILS

FOOD / MEDICATION

Food / Drinks

Meds / Supplements	Time	Dose

☐ usual daily medication

Notes

I am grateful for...

M T W T F S S   DATE:

HOW ARE YOU Feeling today?

😍 Amazing!	🙂 Meh
😁 Great	😠 Not good
🙂 Good	😫 Terrible!

RATE YOUR PAIN LEVEL

① ② ③ ④ ⑤ ⑥ ⑦ ⑧ ⑨ ⑩

WHAT ABOUT YOUR...?

Mood	① ② ③ ④ ⑤ ⑥ ⑦ ⑧ ⑨ ⑩
Energy Levels	① ② ③ ④ ⑤ ⑥ ⑦ ⑧ ⑨ ⑩
Mental Clarity	① ② ③ ④ ⑤ ⑥ ⑦ ⑧ ⑨ ⑩

PAIN & SYMPTOM DETAILS

	am	pm	front	back	other
	☐	☐			☐ Nausea
	☐	☐			☐ Diarrhea
	☐	☐			☐ Vomiting
	☐	☐			☐ Sore throat
	☐	☐			☐ Congestion
	☐	☐			☐ Coughing
	☐	☐			☐ Chills
	☐	☐			☐ Fever

SLEEP

hours _____   quality ① ② ③ ④ ⑤

STRESS LEVELS

None	Low	Medium	High	Max	@$#%!

WEATHER

☐ Cold   ☐ Mild   ☐ Hot
☐ Dry   ☐ Humid   ☐ Wet
Allergen Levels: _____
BM Pressure: _____

EXERCISE

☐ Heck yes, I worked out.
☐ I managed to exercise a bit.
☐ No, I haven't exercised at all.
☐ I did some stuff, and that counts.

DETAILS

FOOD / MEDICATION

Food / Drinks

Meds / Supplements	Time	Dose

☐ usual daily medication

Notes
_____
_____

I am grateful for...

M T W T F S S   DATE:

HOW ARE YOU Feeling today?

Amazing!	Meh
Great	Not good
Good	Terrible!

RATE YOUR PAIN LEVEL

① ② ③ ④ ⑤ ⑥ ⑦ ⑧ ⑨ ⑩

WHAT ABOUT YOUR...?

Mood	① ② ③ ④ ⑤ ⑥ ⑦ ⑧ ⑨ ⑩
Energy Levels	① ② ③ ④ ⑤ ⑥ ⑦ ⑧ ⑨ ⑩
Mental Clarity	① ② ③ ④ ⑤ ⑥ ⑦ ⑧ ⑨ ⑩

PAIN & SYMPTOM DETAILS

	am	pm	*front*	*back*	*other*
_____	☐	☐			☐ Nausea
_____	☐	☐			☐ Diarrhea
_____	☐	☐			☐ Vomiting
_____	☐	☐			☐ Sore throat
_____	☐	☐			☐ Congestion
_____	☐	☐			☐ Coughing
_____	☐	☐			☐ Chills
_____	☐	☐			☐ Fever

SLEEP

hours
_____

quality
① ② ③ ④ ⑤

STRESS LEVELS

None	Low	Medium	High	Max	@$#%!

WEATHER

☐ Cold   ☐ Mild   ☐ Hot
☐ Dry   ☐ Humid   ☐ Wet
Allergen Levels: _____
BM Pressure: _____

EXERCISE

☐ Heck yes, I worked out.
☐ I managed to exercise a bit.
☐ No, I haven't exercised at all.
☐ I did some stuff, and that counts.

DETAILS

FOOD / MEDICATION

Food / Drinks	Meds / Supplements	Time	Dose

☐ usual daily medication

Notes
_____

I am grateful for...
_____

HOW ARE YOU *Feeling today?*

Amazing!	Meh
Great	Not good
Good	Terrible!

RATE YOUR PAIN LEVEL

① ② ③ ④ ⑤ ⑥ ⑦ ⑧ ⑨ ⑩

WHAT ABOUT YOUR...?

Mood	① ② ③ ④ ⑤ ⑥ ⑦ ⑧ ⑨ ⑩
Energy Levels	① ② ③ ④ ⑤ ⑥ ⑦ ⑧ ⑨ ⑩
Mental Clarity	① ② ③ ④ ⑤ ⑥ ⑦ ⑧ ⑨ ⑩

PAIN & SYMPTOM DETAILS

	am	pm	*front*	*back*	*other*
_____	☐	☐			☐ Nausea
_____	☐	☐			☐ Diarrhea
_____	☐	☐			☐ Vomiting
_____	☐	☐			☐ Sore throat
_____	☐	☐			☐ Congestion
_____	☐	☐			☐ Coughing
_____	☐	☐			☐ Chills
_____	☐	☐			☐ Fever

SLEEP

hours
_____

quality
① ② ③ ④ ⑤

STRESS LEVELS

None	Low	Medium	High	Max	@$#%!

WEATHER

☐ Cold ☐ Mild ☐ Hot
☐ Dry ☐ Humid ☐ Wet
Allergen Levels: _____
BM Pressure: _____

EXERCISE

☐ Heck yes, I worked out.
☐ I managed to exercise a bit.
☐ No, I haven't exercised at all.
☐ I did some stuff, and that counts.

DETAILS

FOOD / MEDICATION

Food / Drinks

Meds / Supplements	Time	Dose

☐ usual daily medication

Notes
_____
_____

I am grateful for...

M T W T F S S   DATE:

HOW ARE YOU Feeling today?

😍 Amazing!	🙂 Meh
😁 Great	😠 Not good
😊 Good	😖 Terrible!

RATE YOUR PAIN LEVEL

① ② ③ ④ ⑤ ⑥ ⑦ ⑧ ⑨ ⑩

WHAT ABOUT YOUR...?

Mood	① ② ③ ④ ⑤ ⑥ ⑦ ⑧ ⑨ ⑩
Energy Levels	① ② ③ ④ ⑤ ⑥ ⑦ ⑧ ⑨ ⑩
Mental Clarity	① ② ③ ④ ⑤ ⑥ ⑦ ⑧ ⑨ ⑩

PAIN & SYMPTOM DETAILS

	am	pm	front	back	other
_____	☐	☐			☐ Nausea
_____	☐	☐			☐ Diarrhea
_____	☐	☐			☐ Vomiting
_____	☐	☐			☐ Sore throat
_____	☐	☐			☐ Congestion
_____	☐	☐			☐ Coughing
_____	☐	☐			☐ Chills
_____	☐	☐			☐ Fever

SLEEP

hours _____   _quality_ ① ② ③ ④ ⑤

STRESS LEVELS

None	Low	Medium	High	Max	@$#%!

WEATHER

☐ Cold   ☐ Mild   ☐ Hot
☐ Dry   ☐ Humid   ☐ Wet
Allergen Levels: _____
BM Pressure: _____

EXERCISE

☐ Heck yes, I worked out.
☐ I managed to exercise a bit.
☐ No, I haven't exercised at all.
☐ I did some stuff, and that counts.

DETAILS

FOOD / MEDICATION

Food / Drinks

Meds / Supplements	Time	Dose

☐ usual daily medication

Notes
_____
_____

I am grateful for...
_____

HOW ARE YOU *Feeling today?*

Amazing!	Meh
Great	Not good
Good	Terrible!

RATE YOUR PAIN LEVEL

(1) (2) (3) (4) (5) (6) (7) (8) (9) (10)

WHAT ABOUT YOUR...?

Mood	(1) (2) (3) (4) (5) (6) (7) (8) (9) (10)
Energy Levels	(1) (2) (3) (4) (5) (6) (7) (8) (9) (10)
Mental Clarity	(1) (2) (3) (4) (5) (6) (7) (8) (9) (10)

PAIN & SYMPTOM DETAILS

	am	pm	*front*	*back*	*other*
....	☐	☐			☐ Nausea
....	☐	☐			☐ Diarrhea
....	☐	☐			☐ Vomiting
....	☐	☐			☐ Sore throat
....	☐	☐			☐ Congestion
....	☐	☐			☐ Coughing
....	☐	☐			☐ Chills
....	☐	☐			☐ Fever

SLEEP

hours
_____

quality
(1) (2) (3) (4) (5)

STRESS LEVELS

None	Low	Medium	High	Max	@$#%!

WEATHER

☐ Cold   ☐ Mild   ☐ Hot
☐ Dry   ☐ Humid ☐ Wet

Allergen Levels: _____
BM Pressure: _____

EXERCISE

☐ Heck yes, I worked out.
☐ I managed to exercise a bit.
☐ No, I haven't exercised at all.
☐ I did some stuff, and that counts.

DETAILS

FOOD / MEDICATION

Food / Drinks

Meds / Supplements	Time	Dose

☐ usual daily medication

Notes

I am grateful for...

HOW ARE YOU *Feeling today?*

😍 Amazing!	🙂 Meh
😁 Great	😠 Not good
😊 Good	😤 Terrible!

RATE YOUR PAIN LEVEL

① ② ③ ④ ⑤ ⑥ ⑦ ⑧ ⑨ ⑩

WHAT ABOUT YOUR...?

Mood	① ② ③ ④ ⑤ ⑥ ⑦ ⑧ ⑨ ⑩
Energy Levels	① ② ③ ④ ⑤ ⑥ ⑦ ⑧ ⑨ ⑩
Mental Clarity	① ② ③ ④ ⑤ ⑥ ⑦ ⑧ ⑨ ⑩

PAIN & SYMPTOM DETAILS

	am	pm	front	back	other
_____	☐	☐			☐ Nausea
_____	☐	☐			☐ Diarrhea
_____	☐	☐			☐ Vomiting
_____	☐	☐			☐ Sore throat
_____	☐	☐			☐ Congestion
_____	☐	☐			☐ Coughing
_____	☐	☐			☐ Chills
_____	☐	☐			☐ Fever

SLEEP

hours _____   *quality* ① ② ③ ④ ⑤

STRESS LEVELS

None	Low	Medium	High	Max	@$#%!

WEATHER

☐ Cold   ☐ Mild   ☐ Hot
☐ Dry   ☐ Humid   ☐ Wet
Allergen Levels: _____
BM Pressure: _____

EXERCISE

☐ Heck yes, I worked out.
☐ I managed to exercise a bit.
☐ No, I haven't exercised at all.
☐ I did some stuff, and that counts.

DETAILS

FOOD / MEDICATION

Food / Drinks

Meds / Supplements	Time	Dose

☐ usual daily medication

Notes
_____
_____

I am grateful for...

HOW ARE YOU *Feeling today?*

😍 Amazing!	🙂 Meh
😁 Great	😠 Not good
🙂 Good	😵 Terrible!

RATE YOUR PAIN LEVEL

① ② ③ ④ ⑤ ⑥ ⑦ ⑧ ⑨ ⑩

WHAT ABOUT YOUR...?

Mood	①	②	③	④	⑤	⑥	⑦	⑧	⑨	⑩
Energy Levels	①	②	③	④	⑤	⑥	⑦	⑧	⑨	⑩
Mental Clarity	①	②	③	④	⑤	⑥	⑦	⑧	⑨	⑩

PAIN & SYMPTOM DETAILS

	am	pm	*front*	*back*	*other*
	☐	☐			☐ Nausea
	☐	☐			☐ Diarrhea
	☐	☐			☐ Vomiting
	☐	☐			☐ Sore throat
	☐	☐			☐ Congestion
	☐	☐			☐ Coughing
	☐	☐			☐ Chills
	☐	☐			☐ Fever

SLEEP

hours
_____

quality
① ② ③ ④ ⑤

STRESS LEVELS

None	Low	Medium	High	Max	@$#%!

WEATHER

☐ Cold   ☐ Mild   ☐ Hot
☐ Dry   ☐ Humid   ☐ Wet

Allergen Levels: _____
BM Pressure: _____

EXERCISE

☐ Heck yes, I worked out.
☐ I managed to exercise a bit.
☐ No, I haven't exercised at all.
☐ I did some stuff, and that counts.

DETAILS

FOOD / MEDICATION

Food / Drinks

Meds / Supplements	Time	Dose

☐ usual daily medication

Notes
_____
_____

I am grateful for…
_____

HOW ARE YOU Feeling today?

Amazing!	Meh
Great	Not good
Good	Terrible!

RATE YOUR PAIN LEVEL

① ② ③ ④ ⑤ ⑥ ⑦ ⑧ ⑨ ⑩

WHAT ABOUT YOUR...?

Mood	① ② ③ ④ ⑤ ⑥ ⑦ ⑧ ⑨ ⑩
Energy Levels	① ② ③ ④ ⑤ ⑥ ⑦ ⑧ ⑨ ⑩
Mental Clarity	① ② ③ ④ ⑤ ⑥ ⑦ ⑧ ⑨ ⑩

PAIN & SYMPTOM DETAILS

	am	pm	front	back	other
	☐	☐			☐ Nausea
	☐	☐			☐ Diarrhea
	☐	☐			☐ Vomiting
	☐	☐			☐ Sore throat
	☐	☐			☐ Congestion
	☐	☐			☐ Coughing
	☐	☐			☐ Chills
	☐	☐			☐ Fever

SLEEP

hours _____   *quality* ① ② ③ ④ ⑤

STRESS LEVELS

None	Low	Medium	High	Max	@$#%!

WEATHER

☐ Cold   ☐ Mild   ☐ Hot
☐ Dry   ☐ Humid   ☐ Wet
Allergen Levels: _____
BM Pressure: _____

EXERCISE

☐ Heck yes, I worked out.
☐ I managed to exercise a bit.
☐ No, I haven't exercised at all.
☐ I did some stuff, and that counts.

DETAILS

FOOD / MEDICATION

Food / Drinks	Meds / Supplements	Time	Dose

☐ usual daily medication

Notes

I am grateful for...

M T W T F S S   DATE:

HOW ARE YOU Feeling today?

Amazing!	Meh
Great	Not good
Good	Terrible!

RATE YOUR PAIN LEVEL

① ② ③ ④ ⑤ ⑥ ⑦ ⑧ ⑨ ⑩

WHAT ABOUT YOUR...?

Mood	① ② ③ ④ ⑤ ⑥ ⑦ ⑧ ⑨ ⑩
Energy Levels	① ② ③ ④ ⑤ ⑥ ⑦ ⑧ ⑨ ⑩
Mental Clarity	① ② ③ ④ ⑤ ⑥ ⑦ ⑧ ⑨ ⑩

PAIN & SYMPTOM DETAILS

	am	pm	*front*	*back*	*other*
_____	☐	☐			☐ Nausea
_____	☐	☐			☐ Diarrhea
_____	☐	☐			☐ Vomiting
_____	☐	☐			☐ Sore throat
_____	☐	☐			☐ Congestion
_____	☐	☐			☐ Coughing
_____	☐	☐			☐ Chills
_____	☐	☐			☐ Fever

SLEEP

hours
_____

quality
① ② ③ ④ ⑤

STRESS LEVELS

| None | Low | Medium | High | Max | @$#%! |

WEATHER

☐ Cold   ☐ Mild   ☐ Hot
☐ Dry   ☐ Humid   ☐ Wet

Allergen Levels: _____
BM Pressure: _____

EXERCISE

☐ Heck yes, I worked out.
☐ I managed to exercise a bit.
☐ No, I haven't exercised at all.
☐ I did some stuff, and that counts.

DETAILS

FOOD / MEDICATION

Food / Drinks

Meds / Supplements	Time	Dose

☐ usual daily medication

Notes
_____
_____

I am grateful for...
_____

M T W T F S S

DATE:

HOW ARE YOU *Feeling today?*

Amazing!	Meh
Great	Not good
Good	Terrible!

RATE YOUR PAIN LEVEL

① ② ③ ④ ⑤ ⑥ ⑦ ⑧ ⑨ ⑩

WHAT ABOUT YOUR...?

Mood	① ② ③ ④ ⑤ ⑥ ⑦ ⑧ ⑨ ⑩
Energy Levels	① ② ③ ④ ⑤ ⑥ ⑦ ⑧ ⑨ ⑩
Mental Clarity	① ② ③ ④ ⑤ ⑥ ⑦ ⑧ ⑨ ⑩

PAIN & SYMPTOM DETAILS

	am	pm	*front*	*back*	*other*
_____	☐	☐			☐ Nausea
_____	☐	☐			☐ Diarrhea
_____	☐	☐			☐ Vomiting
_____	☐	☐			☐ Sore throat
_____	☐	☐			☐ Congestion
_____	☐	☐			☐ Coughing
_____	☐	☐			☐ Chills
_____	☐	☐			☐ Fever

SLEEP

hours _____   *quality* ① ② ③ ④ ⑤

STRESS LEVELS

None	Low	Medium	High	Max	@$#%!

WEATHER

☐ Cold   ☐ Mild   ☐ Hot
☐ Dry   ☐ Humid   ☐ Wet
Allergen Levels: _____
BM Pressure: _____

EXERCISE

☐ Heck yes, I worked out.
☐ I managed to exercise a bit.
☐ No, I haven't exercised at all.
☐ I did some stuff, and that counts.

DETAILS

FOOD / MEDICATION

Food / Drinks	Meds / Supplements	Time	Dose

☐ usual daily medication

Notes
_____
_____

I am grateful for...

M T W T F S S

DATE:

HOW ARE YOU *Feeling today?*

😍 Amazing!	🙂 Meh
😁 Great	😠 Not good
🙂 Good	😖 Terrible!

RATE YOUR PAIN LEVEL

① ② ③ ④ ⑤ ⑥ ⑦ ⑧ ⑨ ⑩

WHAT ABOUT YOUR...?

Mood	① ② ③ ④ ⑤ ⑥ ⑦ ⑧ ⑨ ⑩
Energy Levels	① ② ③ ④ ⑤ ⑥ ⑦ ⑧ ⑨ ⑩
Mental Clarity	① ② ③ ④ ⑤ ⑥ ⑦ ⑧ ⑨ ⑩

PAIN & SYMPTOM DETAILS

	am	pm	front	back	other
_____	☐	☐			☐ Nausea
_____	☐	☐			☐ Diarrhea
_____	☐	☐			☐ Vomiting
_____	☐	☐			☐ Sore throat
_____	☐	☐			☐ Congestion
_____	☐	☐			☐ Coughing
_____	☐	☐			☐ Chills
_____	☐	☐			☐ Fever

SLEEP

hours
_____

quality
① ② ③ ④ ⑤

STRESS LEVELS

None	Low	Medium	High	Max	@$#%!

WEATHER

☐ Cold   ☐ Mild   ☐ Hot
☐ Dry   ☐ Humid   ☐ Wet

Allergen Levels: _____
BM Pressure: _____

EXERCISE

☐ Heck yes, I worked out.
☐ I managed to exercise a bit.
☐ No, I haven't exercised at all.
☐ I did some stuff, and that counts.

DETAILS

FOOD / MEDICATION

Food / Drinks

Meds / Supplements	Time	Dose

☐ usual daily medication

Notes
_____
_____

I am grateful for...

M T W T F S S   DATE:

HOW ARE YOU Feeling today?

Amazing!	Meh
Great	Not good
Good	Terrible!

RATE YOUR PAIN LEVEL

① ② ③ ④ ⑤ ⑥ ⑦ ⑧ ⑨ ⑩

WHAT ABOUT YOUR...?

Mood	① ② ③ ④ ⑤ ⑥ ⑦ ⑧ ⑨ ⑩
Energy Levels	① ② ③ ④ ⑤ ⑥ ⑦ ⑧ ⑨ ⑩
Mental Clarity	① ② ③ ④ ⑤ ⑥ ⑦ ⑧ ⑨ ⑩

PAIN & SYMPTOM DETAILS

| | am | pm | front | back | other |

other
- ☐ Nausea
- ☐ Diarrhea
- ☐ Vomiting
- ☐ Sore throat
- ☐ Congestion
- ☐ Coughing
- ☐ Chills
- ☐ Fever

SLEEP

hours _____   quality ① ② ③ ④ ⑤

STRESS LEVELS

| None | Low | Medium | High | Max | @$#%! |

WEATHER

- ☐ Cold ☐ Mild ☐ Hot
- ☐ Dry ☐ Humid ☐ Wet

Allergen Levels: _____

BM Pressure: _____

EXERCISE

- ☐ Heck yes, I worked out.
- ☐ I managed to exercise a bit.
- ☐ No, I haven't exercised at all.
- ☐ I did some stuff, and that counts.

DETAILS

FOOD / MEDICATION

Food / Drinks

Meds / Supplements	Time	Dose

☐ usual daily medication

Notes

I am grateful for…

HOW ARE YOU *Feeling today?*

😍 Amazing!	🙂 Meh
😁 Great	😠 Not good
🙂 Good	😖 Terrible!

RATE YOUR PAIN LEVEL

① ② ③ ④ ⑤ ⑥ ⑦ ⑧ ⑨ ⑩

WHAT ABOUT YOUR...?

Mood	① ② ③ ④ ⑤ ⑥ ⑦ ⑧ ⑨ ⑩
Energy Levels	① ② ③ ④ ⑤ ⑥ ⑦ ⑧ ⑨ ⑩
Mental Clarity	① ② ③ ④ ⑤ ⑥ ⑦ ⑧ ⑨ ⑩

PAIN & SYMPTOM DETAILS

	am	pm	*front*	*back*	*other*
_____	☐	☐			☐ Nausea
_____	☐	☐			☐ Diarrhea
_____	☐	☐			☐ Vomiting
_____	☐	☐			☐ Sore throat
_____	☐	☐			☐ Congestion
_____	☐	☐			☐ Coughing
_____	☐	☐			☐ Chills
_____	☐	☐			☐ Fever

SLEEP

hours _____

quality ① ② ③ ④ ⑤

STRESS LEVELS

None	Low	Medium	High	Max	@$#%!

WEATHER

☐ Cold   ☐ Mild   ☐ Hot
☐ Dry   ☐ Humid   ☐ Wet
Allergen Levels: _____
BM Pressure: _____

EXERCISE

☐ Heck yes, I worked out.
☐ I managed to exercise a bit.
☐ No, I haven't exercised at all.
☐ I did some stuff, and that counts.

DETAILS

FOOD / MEDICATION

Food / Drinks

Meds / Supplements	Time	Dose

☐ usual daily medication

Notes
_____
_____

I am grateful for...

M T W T F S S   DATE:

HOW ARE YOU *Feeling today?*

😍 Amazing!	🙂 Meh
😁 Great	😠 Not good
😊 Good	😖 Terrible!

RATE YOUR PAIN LEVEL

① ② ③ ④ ⑤ ⑥ ⑦ ⑧ ⑨ ⑩

WHAT ABOUT YOUR...?

Mood	① ② ③ ④ ⑤ ⑥ ⑦ ⑧ ⑨ ⑩
Energy Levels	① ② ③ ④ ⑤ ⑥ ⑦ ⑧ ⑨ ⑩
Mental Clarity	① ② ③ ④ ⑤ ⑥ ⑦ ⑧ ⑨ ⑩

PAIN & SYMPTOM DETAILS

	am	pm	front	back	other
	☐	☐			☐ Nausea
	☐	☐			☐ Diarrhea
	☐	☐			☐ Vomiting
	☐	☐			☐ Sore throat
	☐	☐			☐ Congestion
	☐	☐			☐ Coughing
	☐	☐			☐ Chills
	☐	☐			☐ Fever

SLEEP

hours _____   *quality* ① ② ③ ④ ⑤

STRESS LEVELS

None	Low	Medium	High	Max	@$#%!

WEATHER

☐ Cold   ☐ Mild   ☐ Hot
☐ Dry   ☐ Humid   ☐ Wet
Allergen Levels: _____
BM Pressure: _____

EXERCISE

☐ Heck yes, I worked out.
☐ I managed to exercise a bit.
☐ No, I haven't exercised at all.
☐ I did some stuff, and that counts.

DETAILS

FOOD / MEDICATION

Food / Drinks

Meds / Supplements	Time	Dose

☐ usual daily medication

Notes

I am grateful for...

HOW ARE YOU
Feeling today?

😍 Amazing!	🙂 Meh
😁 Great	😠 Not good
😊 Good	😖 Terrible!

RATE YOUR PAIN LEVEL

① ② ③ ④ ⑤ ⑥ ⑦ ⑧ ⑨ ⑩

WHAT ABOUT YOUR...?

Mood	① ② ③ ④ ⑤ ⑥ ⑦ ⑧ ⑨ ⑩
Energy Levels	① ② ③ ④ ⑤ ⑥ ⑦ ⑧ ⑨ ⑩
Mental Clarity	① ② ③ ④ ⑤ ⑥ ⑦ ⑧ ⑨ ⑩

PAIN & SYMPTOM DETAILS

	am	pm		other
_____	☐	☐	*front* *back*	☐ Nausea
_____	☐	☐		☐ Diarrhea
_____	☐	☐		☐ Vomiting
_____	☐	☐		☐ Sore throat
_____	☐	☐		☐ Congestion
_____	☐	☐		☐ Coughing
_____	☐	☐		☐ Chills
_____	☐	☐		☐ Fever

SLEEP

hours
_____

quality
① ② ③ ④ ⑤

STRESS LEVELS

None	Low	Medium	High	Max	@$#%!

WEATHER

☐ Cold   ☐ Mild   ☐ Hot
☐ Dry   ☐ Humid   ☐ Wet
Allergen Levels: _____
BM Pressure: _____

EXERCISE

☐ Heck yes, I worked out.
☐ I managed to exercise a bit.
☐ No, I haven't exercised at all.
☐ I did some stuff, and that counts.

DETAILS

FOOD / MEDICATION

Food / Drinks

Meds / Supplements	Time	Dose

☐ usual daily medication

Notes
_____
_____

I am grateful for…

HOW ARE YOU *Feeling today?*

😊 Amazing!	🙂 Meh
😁 Great	😣 Not good
🙂 Good	😵 Terrible!

RATE YOUR PAIN LEVEL

① ② ③ ④ ⑤ ⑥ ⑦ ⑧ ⑨ ⑩

WHAT ABOUT YOUR...?

Mood	① ② ③ ④ ⑤ ⑥ ⑦ ⑧ ⑨ ⑩
Energy Levels	① ② ③ ④ ⑤ ⑥ ⑦ ⑧ ⑨ ⑩
Mental Clarity	① ② ③ ④ ⑤ ⑥ ⑦ ⑧ ⑨ ⑩

PAIN & SYMPTOM DETAILS

	am	pm	*front*	*back*	*other*
_____	☐	☐			☐ Nausea
_____	☐	☐			☐ Diarrhea
_____	☐	☐			☐ Vomiting
_____	☐	☐			☐ Sore throat
_____	☐	☐			☐ Congestion
_____	☐	☐			☐ Coughing
_____	☐	☐			☐ Chills
_____	☐	☐			☐ Fever

SLEEP

hours   *quality*
_____   ① ② ③ ④ ⑤

STRESS LEVELS

None	Low	Medium	High	Max	@$#%!

WEATHER

☐ Cold   ☐ Mild   ☐ Hot
☐ Dry   ☐ Humid ☐ Wet
Allergen Levels: _____
BM Pressure: _____

EXERCISE

☐ Heck yes, I worked out.
☐ I managed to exercise a bit.
☐ No, I haven't exercised at all.
☐ I did some stuff, and that counts.

DETAILS

FOOD / MEDICATION

Food / Drinks

Meds / Supplements	Time	Dose

☐ usual daily medication

Notes
_____
_____

I am grateful for...

M T W T F S S   DATE:

HOW ARE YOU Feeling today?

☺ Amazing!	😐 Meh
😁 Great	😠 Not good
🙂 Good	😫 Terrible!

RATE YOUR PAIN LEVEL

① ② ③ ④ ⑤ ⑥ ⑦ ⑧ ⑨ ⑩

WHAT ABOUT YOUR...?

Mood	① ② ③ ④ ⑤ ⑥ ⑦ ⑧ ⑨ ⑩
Energy Levels	① ② ③ ④ ⑤ ⑥ ⑦ ⑧ ⑨ ⑩
Mental Clarity	① ② ③ ④ ⑤ ⑥ ⑦ ⑧ ⑨ ⑩

PAIN & SYMPTOM DETAILS

	am	pm	front	back	other
	☐	☐			☐ Nausea
	☐	☐			☐ Diarrhea
	☐	☐			☐ Vomiting
	☐	☐			☐ Sore throat
	☐	☐			☐ Congestion
	☐	☐			☐ Coughing
	☐	☐			☐ Chills
	☐	☐			☐ Fever

SLEEP

hours _____

quality ① ② ③ ④ ⑤

STRESS LEVELS

None	Low	Medium	High	Max	@$#%!

WEATHER

☐ Cold ☐ Mild ☐ Hot
☐ Dry ☐ Humid ☐ Wet
Allergen Levels: _____
BM Pressure: _____

EXERCISE

☐ Heck yes, I worked out.
☐ I managed to exercise a bit.
☐ No, I haven't exercised at all.
☐ I did some stuff, and that counts.

DETAILS

FOOD / MEDICATION

Food / Drinks

Meds / Supplements	Time	Dose

☐ usual daily medication

Notes

I am grateful for...

HOW ARE YOU *Feeling today?*

😍 Amazing!	🙂 Meh
😁 Great	😠 Not good
😊 Good	😣 Terrible!

RATE YOUR PAIN LEVEL

① ② ③ ④ ⑤ ⑥ ⑦ ⑧ ⑨ ⑩

WHAT ABOUT YOUR...?

Mood	① ② ③ ④ ⑤ ⑥ ⑦ ⑧ ⑨ ⑩
Energy Levels	① ② ③ ④ ⑤ ⑥ ⑦ ⑧ ⑨ ⑩
Mental Clarity	① ② ③ ④ ⑤ ⑥ ⑦ ⑧ ⑨ ⑩

PAIN & SYMPTOM DETAILS

	am	pm	front	back	other
_____	☐	☐			☐ Nausea
_____	☐	☐			☐ Diarrhea
_____	☐	☐			☐ Vomiting
_____	☐	☐			☐ Sore throat
_____	☐	☐			☐ Congestion
_____	☐	☐			☐ Coughing
_____	☐	☐			☐ Chills
_____	☐	☐			☐ Fever

SLEEP

hours _____   *quality* ① ② ③ ④ ⑤

STRESS LEVELS

None	Low	Medium	High	Max	@$#%!

WEATHER

☐ Cold   ☐ Mild   ☐ Hot
☐ Dry   ☐ Humid   ☐ Wet
Allergen Levels: _____
BM Pressure: _____

EXERCISE

☐ Heck yes, I worked out.
☐ I managed to exercise a bit.
☐ No, I haven't exercised at all.
☐ I did some stuff, and that counts.

DETAILS

FOOD / MEDICATION

Food / Drinks

Meds / Supplements	Time	Dose

☐ usual daily medication

Notes
_____
_____

I am grateful for...

M T W T F S S   DATE:

HOW ARE YOU *Feeling today?*

Amazing!	Meh
Great	Not good
Good	Terrible!

RATE YOUR PAIN LEVEL

① ② ③ ④ ⑤ ⑥ ⑦ ⑧ ⑨ ⑩

WHAT ABOUT YOUR...?

Mood	① ② ③ ④ ⑤ ⑥ ⑦ ⑧ ⑨ ⑩
Energy Levels	① ② ③ ④ ⑤ ⑥ ⑦ ⑧ ⑨ ⑩
Mental Clarity	① ② ③ ④ ⑤ ⑥ ⑦ ⑧ ⑨ ⑩

PAIN & SYMPTOM DETAILS

	am	pm	front	back	other
	☐	☐			☐ Nausea
	☐	☐			☐ Diarrhea
	☐	☐			☐ Vomiting
	☐	☐			☐ Sore throat
	☐	☐			☐ Congestion
	☐	☐			☐ Coughing
	☐	☐			☐ Chills
	☐	☐			☐ Fever

SLEEP

hours _____

quality ① ② ③ ④ ⑤

STRESS LEVELS

| None | Low | Medium | High | Max | @$#%! |

WEATHER

☐ Cold   ☐ Mild   ☐ Hot
☐ Dry   ☐ Humid   ☐ Wet
Allergen Levels: _____
BM Pressure: _____

EXERCISE

☐ Heck yes, I worked out.
☐ I managed to exercise a bit.
☐ No, I haven't exercised at all.
☐ I did some stuff, and that counts.

DETAILS

FOOD / MEDICATION

Food / Drinks

Meds / Supplements	Time	Dose

☐ usual daily medication

Notes
_____
_____

I am grateful for...
_____

M T W T F S S

DATE:

HOW ARE YOU *Feeling today?*

Amazing!	Meh
Great	Not good
Good	Terrible!

RATE YOUR PAIN LEVEL

① ② ③ ④ ⑤ ⑥ ⑦ ⑧ ⑨ ⑩

WHAT ABOUT YOUR...?

Mood	① ② ③ ④ ⑤ ⑥ ⑦ ⑧ ⑨ ⑩
Energy Levels	① ② ③ ④ ⑤ ⑥ ⑦ ⑧ ⑨ ⑩
Mental Clarity	① ② ③ ④ ⑤ ⑥ ⑦ ⑧ ⑨ ⑩

PAIN & SYMPTOM DETAILS

	am	pm	front	back	other
	☐	☐			☐ Nausea
	☐	☐			☐ Diarrhea
	☐	☐			☐ Vomiting
	☐	☐			☐ Sore throat
	☐	☐			☐ Congestion
	☐	☐			☐ Coughing
	☐	☐			☐ Chills
	☐	☐			☐ Fever

SLEEP

hours
_____

quality
① ② ③ ④ ⑤

STRESS LEVELS

None	Low	Medium	High	Max	@$#%!

WEATHER

☐ Cold   ☐ Mild   ☐ Hot
☐ Dry   ☐ Humid   ☐ Wet

Allergen Levels: _____
BM Pressure: _____

EXERCISE

☐ Heck yes, I worked out.
☐ I managed to exercise a bit.
☐ No, I haven't exercised at all.
☐ I did some stuff, and that counts.

DETAILS

FOOD / MEDICATION

Food / Drinks

Meds / Supplements	Time	Dose

☐ usual daily medication

Notes
_____
_____

I am grateful for...

HOW ARE YOU *Feeling today?*

😍 Amazing!	🙂 Meh
😁 Great	😠 Not good
😊 Good	😣 Terrible!

RATE YOUR PAIN LEVEL

① ② ③ ④ ⑤ ⑥ ⑦ ⑧ ⑨ ⑩

WHAT ABOUT YOUR...?

Mood	① ② ③ ④ ⑤ ⑥ ⑦ ⑧ ⑨ ⑩
Energy Levels	① ② ③ ④ ⑤ ⑥ ⑦ ⑧ ⑨ ⑩
Mental Clarity	① ② ③ ④ ⑤ ⑥ ⑦ ⑧ ⑨ ⑩

PAIN & SYMPTOM DETAILS

	am	pm	*front*	*back*	*other*
_____	☐	☐			☐ Nausea
_____	☐	☐			☐ Diarrhea
_____	☐	☐			☐ Vomiting
_____	☐	☐			☐ Sore throat
_____	☐	☐			☐ Congestion
_____	☐	☐			☐ Coughing
_____	☐	☐			☐ Chills
_____	☐	☐			☐ Fever

SLEEP

hours _____

quality ① ② ③ ④ ⑤

STRESS LEVELS

None	Low	Medium	High	Max	@$#%!

WEATHER

☐ Cold   ☐ Mild   ☐ Hot
☐ Dry   ☐ Humid   ☐ Wet

Allergen Levels: _____
BM Pressure: _____

EXERCISE

☐ Heck yes, I worked out.
☐ I managed to exercise a bit.
☐ No, I haven't exercised at all.
☐ I did some stuff, and that counts.

DETAILS

FOOD / MEDICATION

Food / Drinks

Meds / Supplements	Time	Dose

☐ usual daily medication

Notes
_____
_____

I am grateful for...

HOW ARE YOU *Feeling today?*

😍 Amazing!	🙂 Meh
😁 Great	😣 Not good
😊 Good	😖 Terrible!

RATE YOUR PAIN LEVEL

① ② ③ ④ ⑤ ⑥ ⑦ ⑧ ⑨ ⑩

WHAT ABOUT YOUR...?

Mood	① ② ③ ④ ⑤ ⑥ ⑦ ⑧ ⑨ ⑩
Energy Levels	① ② ③ ④ ⑤ ⑥ ⑦ ⑧ ⑨ ⑩
Mental Clarity	① ② ③ ④ ⑤ ⑥ ⑦ ⑧ ⑨ ⑩

PAIN & SYMPTOM DETAILS

	am	pm
	☐	☐
	☐	☐
	☐	☐
	☐	☐
	☐	☐
	☐	☐
	☐	☐
	☐	☐

front   *back*

other
- ☐ Nausea
- ☐ Diarrhea
- ☐ Vomiting
- ☐ Sore throat
- ☐ Congestion
- ☐ Coughing
- ☐ Chills
- ☐ Fever

SLEEP

hours _____   *quality* ① ② ③ ④ ⑤

STRESS LEVELS

None	Low	Medium	High	Max	@$#%!

WEATHER

☐ Cold   ☐ Mild   ☐ Hot
☐ Dry   ☐ Humid   ☐ Wet

Allergen Levels: _____
BM Pressure: _____

EXERCISE

☐ Heck yes, I worked out.
☐ I managed to exercise a bit.
☐ No, I haven't exercised at all.
☐ I did some stuff, and that counts.

DETAILS

FOOD / MEDICATION

Food / Drinks

Meds / Supplements	Time	Dose

☐ usual daily medication

Notes

I am grateful for...

M T W T F S S

DATE:

HOW ARE YOU *Feeling today?*

Amazing!	Meh
Great	Not good
Good	Terrible!

RATE YOUR PAIN LEVEL

① ② ③ ④ ⑤ ⑥ ⑦ ⑧ ⑨ ⑩

WHAT ABOUT YOUR...?

Mood	① ② ③ ④ ⑤ ⑥ ⑦ ⑧ ⑨ ⑩
Energy Levels	① ② ③ ④ ⑤ ⑥ ⑦ ⑧ ⑨ ⑩
Mental Clarity	① ② ③ ④ ⑤ ⑥ ⑦ ⑧ ⑨ ⑩

PAIN & SYMPTOM DETAILS

	am	pm	*front*	*back*	*other*
_____	☐	☐			☐ Nausea
_____	☐	☐			☐ Diarrhea
_____	☐	☐			☐ Vomiting
_____	☐	☐			☐ Sore throat
_____	☐	☐			☐ Congestion
_____	☐	☐			☐ Coughing
_____	☐	☐			☐ Chills
_____	☐	☐			☐ Fever

SLEEP

hours
_____

quality
① ② ③ ④ ⑤

STRESS LEVELS

None	Low	Medium	High	Max	@$#%!

WEATHER

☐ Cold ☐ Mild ☐ Hot
☐ Dry ☐ Humid ☐ Wet
Allergen Levels: _____
BM Pressure: _____

EXERCISE

☐ Heck yes, I worked out.
☐ I managed to exercise a bit.
☐ No, I haven't exercised at all.
☐ I did some stuff, and that counts.

DETAILS

FOOD / MEDICATION

Food / Drinks

Meds / Supplements	Time	Dose

☐ usual daily medication

Notes

_____

I am grateful for…

M T W T F S S   DATE:

HOW ARE YOU Feeling today?

😍 Amazing!	🙂 Meh
😁 Great	😣 Not good
😊 Good	😵 Terrible!

RATE YOUR PAIN LEVEL
① ② ③ ④ ⑤ ⑥ ⑦ ⑧ ⑨ ⑩

WHAT ABOUT YOUR...?

Mood	① ② ③ ④ ⑤ ⑥ ⑦ ⑧ ⑨ ⑩
Energy Levels	① ② ③ ④ ⑤ ⑥ ⑦ ⑧ ⑨ ⑩
Mental Clarity	① ② ③ ④ ⑤ ⑥ ⑦ ⑧ ⑨ ⑩

PAIN & SYMPTOM DETAILS

	am	pm	front	back	other
_____	☐	☐			☐ Nausea
_____	☐	☐			☐ Diarrhea
_____	☐	☐			☐ Vomiting
_____	☐	☐			☐ Sore throat
_____	☐	☐			☐ Congestion
_____	☐	☐			☐ Coughing
_____	☐	☐			☐ Chills
_____	☐	☐			☐ Fever

SLEEP

hours   quality
_____   ① ② ③ ④ ⑤

STRESS LEVELS

None	Low	Medium	High	Max	@$#%!

WEATHER

☐ Cold   ☐ Mild   ☐ Hot
☐ Dry   ☐ Humid   ☐ Wet
Allergen Levels: _____
BM Pressure: _____

EXERCISE

☐ Heck yes, I worked out.
☐ I managed to exercise a bit.
☐ No, I haven't exercised at all.
☐ I did some stuff, and that counts.

DETAILS

FOOD / MEDICATION

Food / Drinks

Meds / Supplements	Time	Dose

☐ usual daily medication

Notes
_____
_____

I am grateful for...

HOW ARE YOU *Feeling today?*

😍 Amazing!	🙂 Meh
😁 Great	😠 Not good
🙂 Good	😖 Terrible!

RATE YOUR PAIN LEVEL

① ② ③ ④ ⑤ ⑥ ⑦ ⑧ ⑨ ⑩

WHAT ABOUT YOUR...?

Mood	① ② ③ ④ ⑤ ⑥ ⑦ ⑧ ⑨ ⑩
Energy Levels	① ② ③ ④ ⑤ ⑥ ⑦ ⑧ ⑨ ⑩
Mental Clarity	① ② ③ ④ ⑤ ⑥ ⑦ ⑧ ⑨ ⑩

PAIN & SYMPTOM DETAILS

	am	pm	*front*	*back*	*other*
_____	☐	☐			☐ Nausea
_____	☐	☐			☐ Diarrhea
_____	☐	☐			☐ Vomiting
_____	☐	☐			☐ Sore throat
_____	☐	☐			☐ Congestion
_____	☐	☐			☐ Coughing
_____	☐	☐			☐ Chills
_____	☐	☐			☐ Fever

SLEEP

hours
_____

quality
① ② ③ ④ ⑤

STRESS LEVELS

None	Low	Medium	High	Max	@$#%!

WEATHER

☐ Cold   ☐ Mild   ☐ Hot
☐ Dry   ☐ Humid   ☐ Wet

Allergen Levels: _____
BM Pressure: _____

EXERCISE

☐ Heck yes, I worked out.
☐ I managed to exercise a bit.
☐ No, I haven't exercised at all.
☐ I did some stuff, and that counts.

DETAILS

FOOD / MEDICATION

Food / Drinks

Meds / Supplements	Time	Dose

☐ usual daily medication

Notes
_____
_____

I am grateful for...

HOW ARE YOU *Feeling today?*

😍 Amazing!	🙂 Meh
😁 Great	😠 Not good
😊 Good	😵 Terrible!

RATE YOUR PAIN LEVEL

① ② ③ ④ ⑤ ⑥ ⑦ ⑧ ⑨ ⑩

WHAT ABOUT YOUR...?

Mood	① ② ③ ④ ⑤ ⑥ ⑦ ⑧ ⑨ ⑩
Energy Levels	① ② ③ ④ ⑤ ⑥ ⑦ ⑧ ⑨ ⑩
Mental Clarity	① ② ③ ④ ⑤ ⑥ ⑦ ⑧ ⑨ ⑩

PAIN & SYMPTOM DETAILS

	am	pm
_____	☐	☐
_____	☐	☐
_____	☐	☐
_____	☐	☐
_____	☐	☐
_____	☐	☐
_____	☐	☐
_____	☐	☐

front   *back*

other

☐ Nausea
☐ Diarrhea
☐ Vomiting
☐ Sore throat
☐ Congestion
☐ Coughing
☐ Chills
☐ Fever

SLEEP

hours
_____

quality
① ② ③ ④ ⑤

STRESS LEVELS

None	Low	Medium	High	Max	@$#%!

WEATHER

☐ Cold   ☐ Mild   ☐ Hot
☐ Dry   ☐ Humid ☐ Wet

Allergen Levels: _____
BM Pressure: _____

EXERCISE

☐ Heck yes, I worked out.
☐ I managed to exercise a bit.
☐ No, I haven't exercised at all.
☐ I did some stuff, and that counts.

DETAILS

FOOD / MEDICATION

Food / Drinks

Meds / Supplements	Time	Dose

☐ usual daily medication

Notes
_____
_____

I am grateful for...

HOW ARE YOU *Feeling today?*

Amazing!	Meh
Great	Not good
Good	Terrible!

RATE YOUR PAIN LEVEL

(1) (2) (3) (4) (5) (6) (7) (8) (9) (10)

WHAT ABOUT YOUR...?

Mood	(1) (2) (3) (4) (5) (6) (7) (8) (9) (10)
Energy Levels	(1) (2) (3) (4) (5) (6) (7) (8) (9) (10)
Mental Clarity	(1) (2) (3) (4) (5) (6) (7) (8) (9) (10)

PAIN & SYMPTOM DETAILS

	am	pm	front	back	other
_____	☐	☐			☐ Nausea
_____	☐	☐			☐ Diarrhea
_____	☐	☐			☐ Vomiting
_____	☐	☐			☐ Sore throat
_____	☐	☐			☐ Congestion
_____	☐	☐			☐ Coughing
_____	☐	☐			☐ Chills
_____	☐	☐			☐ Fever

SLEEP

hours _____   *quality* (1) (2) (3) (4) (5)

STRESS LEVELS

None	Low	Medium	High	Max	@$#%!

WEATHER

☐ Cold   ☐ Mild   ☐ Hot
☐ Dry   ☐ Humid   ☐ Wet
Allergen Levels: _____
BM Pressure: _____

EXERCISE

☐ Heck yes, I worked out.
☐ I managed to exercise a bit.
☐ No, I haven't exercised at all.
☐ I did some stuff, and that counts.

DETAILS

FOOD / MEDICATION

Food / Drinks

Meds / Supplements	Time	Dose

☐ usual daily medication

Notes
_____
_____

I am grateful for...
_____

M T W T F S S   DATE:

HOW ARE YOU Feeling today?

Amazing!	Meh
Great	Not good
Good	Terrible!

RATE YOUR PAIN LEVEL

(1) (2) (3) (4) (5) (6) (7) (8) (9) (10)

WHAT ABOUT YOUR...?

Mood	(1) (2) (3) (4) (5) (6) (7) (8) (9) (10)
Energy Levels	(1) (2) (3) (4) (5) (6) (7) (8) (9) (10)
Mental Clarity	(1) (2) (3) (4) (5) (6) (7) (8) (9) (10)

PAIN & SYMPTOM DETAILS

	am	pm	front	back	other
	☐	☐			☐ Nausea
	☐	☐			☐ Diarrhea
	☐	☐			☐ Vomiting
	☐	☐			☐ Sore throat
	☐	☐			☐ Congestion
	☐	☐			☐ Coughing
	☐	☐			☐ Chills
	☐	☐			☐ Fever

SLEEP

hours _____   quality (1) (2) (3) (4) (5)

STRESS LEVELS

None	Low	Medium	High	Max	@$#%!

WEATHER

☐ Cold   ☐ Mild   ☐ Hot
☐ Dry   ☐ Humid   ☐ Wet
Allergen Levels: _____
BM Pressure: _____

EXERCISE

☐ Heck yes, I worked out.
☐ I managed to exercise a bit.
☐ No, I haven't exercised at all.
☐ I did some stuff, and that counts.

DETAILS

FOOD / MEDICATION

Food / Drinks

Meds / Supplements	Time	Dose

☐ usual daily medication

Notes
_____
_____

I am grateful for...
_____

HOW ARE YOU Feeling today?

Amazing!	Meh
Great	Not good
Good	Terrible!

RATE YOUR PAIN LEVEL

① ② ③ ④ ⑤ ⑥ ⑦ ⑧ ⑨ ⑩

WHAT ABOUT YOUR...?

Mood	① ② ③ ④ ⑤ ⑥ ⑦ ⑧ ⑨ ⑩
Energy Levels	① ② ③ ④ ⑤ ⑥ ⑦ ⑧ ⑨ ⑩
Mental Clarity	① ② ③ ④ ⑤ ⑥ ⑦ ⑧ ⑨ ⑩

PAIN & SYMPTOM DETAILS

	am	pm	front	back	other
_____	☐	☐			☐ Nausea
_____	☐	☐			☐ Diarrhea
_____	☐	☐			☐ Vomiting
_____	☐	☐			☐ Sore throat
_____	☐	☐			☐ Congestion
_____	☐	☐			☐ Coughing
_____	☐	☐			☐ Chills
_____	☐	☐			☐ Fever

SLEEP

hours
_____

quality
① ② ③ ④ ⑤

STRESS LEVELS

None	Low	Medium	High	Max	@$#%!

WEATHER

☐ Cold   ☐ Mild   ☐ Hot
☐ Dry   ☐ Humid   ☐ Wet
Allergen Levels: _____
BM Pressure: _____

EXERCISE

☐ Heck yes, I worked out.
☐ I managed to exercise a bit.
☐ No, I haven't exercised at all.
☐ I did some stuff, and that counts.

DETAILS

FOOD / MEDICATION

Food / Drinks

Meds / Supplements	Time	Dose

☐ usual daily medication

Notes
_____
_____

I am grateful for...

M T W T F S S   DATE:

RATE YOUR PAIN LEVEL

① ② ③ ④ ⑤ ⑥ ⑦ ⑧ ⑨ ⑩

HOW ARE YOU *Feeling today?*

😍 Amazing!	🙂 Meh
😁 Great	😣 Not good
😊 Good	😫 Terrible!

WHAT ABOUT YOUR...?

Mood	① ② ③ ④ ⑤ ⑥ ⑦ ⑧ ⑨ ⑩
Energy Levels	① ② ③ ④ ⑤ ⑥ ⑦ ⑧ ⑨ ⑩
Mental Clarity	① ② ③ ④ ⑤ ⑥ ⑦ ⑧ ⑨ ⑩

PAIN & SYMPTOM DETAILS

	am	pm	*front*	*back*	*other*
_____	☐	☐			☐ Nausea
_____	☐	☐			☐ Diarrhea
_____	☐	☐			☐ Vomiting
_____	☐	☐			☐ Sore throat
_____	☐	☐			☐ Congestion
_____	☐	☐			☐ Coughing
_____	☐	☐			☐ Chills
_____	☐	☐			☐ Fever

SLEEP

hours
_____

quality
① ② ③ ④ ⑤

STRESS LEVELS

None	Low	Medium	High	Max	@$#%!

WEATHER

☐ Cold   ☐ Mild   ☐ Hot
☐ Dry   ☐ Humid   ☐ Wet

Allergen Levels: _____
BM Pressure: _____

EXERCISE

☐ Heck yes, I worked out.
☐ I managed to exercise a bit.
☐ No, I haven't exercised at all.
☐ I did some stuff, and that counts.

DETAILS

FOOD / MEDICATION

Food / Drinks

Meds / Supplements	Time	Dose

☐ usual daily medication

Notes
_____
_____

I am grateful for...

HOW ARE YOU *Feeling today?*

Amazing!	Meh
Great	Not good
Good	Terrible!

RATE YOUR PAIN LEVEL

① ② ③ ④ ⑤ ⑥ ⑦ ⑧ ⑨ ⑩

WHAT ABOUT YOUR...?

Mood	① ② ③ ④ ⑤ ⑥ ⑦ ⑧ ⑨ ⑩
Energy Levels	① ② ③ ④ ⑤ ⑥ ⑦ ⑧ ⑨ ⑩
Mental Clarity	① ② ③ ④ ⑤ ⑥ ⑦ ⑧ ⑨ ⑩

PAIN & SYMPTOM DETAILS

	am	pm	front	back	other
	☐	☐			☐ Nausea
	☐	☐			☐ Diarrhea
	☐	☐			☐ Vomiting
	☐	☐			☐ Sore throat
	☐	☐			☐ Congestion
	☐	☐			☐ Coughing
	☐	☐			☐ Chills
	☐	☐			☐ Fever

SLEEP

hours _____   *quality* ① ② ③ ④ ⑤

STRESS LEVELS

None	Low	Medium	High	Max	@$#%!

WEATHER

☐ Cold　☐ Mild　☐ Hot
☐ Dry　☐ Humid　☐ Wet
Allergen Levels: _____
BM Pressure: _____

EXERCISE

☐ Heck yes, I worked out.
☐ I managed to exercise a bit.
☐ No, I haven't exercised at all.
☐ I did some stuff, and that counts.

DETAILS

FOOD / MEDICATION

Food / Drinks

Meds / Supplements	Time	Dose

☐ usual daily medication

Notes

I am grateful for...

HOW ARE YOU *Feeling today?*

Amazing!	Meh
Great	Not good
Good	Terrible!

RATE YOUR PAIN LEVEL

① ② ③ ④ ⑤ ⑥ ⑦ ⑧ ⑨ ⑩

WHAT ABOUT YOUR...?

Mood	① ② ③ ④ ⑤ ⑥ ⑦ ⑧ ⑨ ⑩
Energy Levels	① ② ③ ④ ⑤ ⑥ ⑦ ⑧ ⑨ ⑩
Mental Clarity	① ② ③ ④ ⑤ ⑥ ⑦ ⑧ ⑨ ⑩

PAIN & SYMPTOM DETAILS

	am	pm	front	back	other
	☐	☐			☐ Nausea
	☐	☐			☐ Diarrhea
	☐	☐			☐ Vomiting
	☐	☐			☐ Sore throat
	☐	☐			☐ Congestion
	☐	☐			☐ Coughing
	☐	☐			☐ Chills
	☐	☐			☐ Fever

SLEEP

hours _____

quality ① ② ③ ④ ⑤

STRESS LEVELS

None	Low	Medium	High	Max	@$#%!

WEATHER

☐ Cold   ☐ Mild   ☐ Hot
☐ Dry   ☐ Humid   ☐ Wet

Allergen Levels: _____
BM Pressure: _____

EXERCISE

☐ Heck yes, I worked out.
☐ I managed to exercise a bit.
☐ No, I haven't exercised at all.
☐ I did some stuff, and that counts.

DETAILS

FOOD / MEDICATION

Food / Drinks	Meds / Supplements	Time	Dose

☐ usual daily medication

Notes

I am grateful for...

M T W T F S S   DATE:

HOW ARE YOU *Feeling today?*

😍 Amazing!	🙂 Meh
😁 Great	😠 Not good
😊 Good	😖 Terrible!

RATE YOUR PAIN LEVEL
① ② ③ ④ ⑤ ⑥ ⑦ ⑧ ⑨ ⑩

WHAT ABOUT YOUR...?

Mood	① ② ③ ④ ⑤ ⑥ ⑦ ⑧ ⑨ ⑩
Energy Levels	① ② ③ ④ ⑤ ⑥ ⑦ ⑧ ⑨ ⑩
Mental Clarity	① ② ③ ④ ⑤ ⑥ ⑦ ⑧ ⑨ ⑩

PAIN & SYMPTOM DETAILS

	am	pm	front	back	other
_____	☐	☐			☐ Nausea
_____	☐	☐			☐ Diarrhea
_____	☐	☐			☐ Vomiting
_____	☐	☐			☐ Sore throat
_____	☐	☐			☐ Congestion
_____	☐	☐			☐ Coughing
_____	☐	☐			☐ Chills
_____	☐	☐			☐ Fever

SLEEP

hours
_____

quality
① ② ③ ④ ⑤

STRESS LEVELS

None	Low	Medium	High	Max	@$#%!

WEATHER

☐ Cold   ☐ Mild   ☐ Hot
☐ Dry   ☐ Humid   ☐ Wet
Allergen Levels: _____
BM Pressure: _____

EXERCISE

☐ Heck yes, I worked out.
☐ I managed to exercise a bit.
☐ No, I haven't exercised at all.
☐ I did some stuff, and that counts.

DETAILS

FOOD / MEDICATION

Food / Drinks

Meds / Supplements	Time	Dose

☐ usual daily medication

Notes
_____

I am grateful for...

M T W T F S S

DATE:

HOW ARE YOU Feeling today?

Amazing!	Meh
Great	Not good
Good	Terrible!

RATE YOUR PAIN LEVEL

(1) (2) (3) (4) (5) (6) (7) (8) (9) (10)

WHAT ABOUT YOUR...?

Mood	(1) (2) (3) (4) (5) (6) (7) (8) (9) (10)
Energy Levels	(1) (2) (3) (4) (5) (6) (7) (8) (9) (10)
Mental Clarity	(1) (2) (3) (4) (5) (6) (7) (8) (9) (10)

PAIN & SYMPTOM DETAILS

	am	pm	front	back	other
	☐	☐			☐ Nausea
	☐	☐			☐ Diarrhea
	☐	☐			☐ Vomiting
	☐	☐			☐ Sore throat
	☐	☐			☐ Congestion
	☐	☐			☐ Coughing
	☐	☐			☐ Chills
	☐	☐			☐ Fever

SLEEP

hours _____

quality (1) (2) (3) (4) (5)

STRESS LEVELS

None	Low	Medium	High	Max	@$#%!

WEATHER

☐ Cold   ☐ Mild   ☐ Hot
☐ Dry   ☐ Humid ☐ Wet

Allergen Levels: _____

BM Pressure: _____

EXERCISE

☐ Heck yes, I worked out.
☐ I managed to exercise a bit.
☐ No, I haven't exercised at all.
☐ I did some stuff, and that counts.

DETAILS

FOOD / MEDICATION

Food / Drinks

Meds / Supplements	Time	Dose

☐ usual daily medication

Notes

I am grateful for...

HOW ARE YOU Feeling today?

Amazing!	Meh
Great	Not good
Good	Terrible!

RATE YOUR PAIN LEVEL

① ② ③ ④ ⑤ ⑥ ⑦ ⑧ ⑨ ⑩

WHAT ABOUT YOUR...?

Mood	① ② ③ ④ ⑤ ⑥ ⑦ ⑧ ⑨ ⑩
Energy Levels	① ② ③ ④ ⑤ ⑥ ⑦ ⑧ ⑨ ⑩
Mental Clarity	① ② ③ ④ ⑤ ⑥ ⑦ ⑧ ⑨ ⑩

PAIN & SYMPTOM DETAILS

	am	pm
	☐	☐
	☐	☐
	☐	☐
	☐	☐
	☐	☐
	☐	☐
	☐	☐
	☐	☐

front *back*

other

- ☐ Nausea
- ☐ Diarrhea
- ☐ Vomiting
- ☐ Sore throat
- ☐ Congestion
- ☐ Coughing
- ☐ Chills
- ☐ Fever

SLEEP

hours _____ *quality* ① ② ③ ④ ⑤

STRESS LEVELS

None	Low	Medium	High	Max	@$#%!

WEATHER

- ☐ Cold   ☐ Mild   ☐ Hot
- ☐ Dry   ☐ Humid   ☐ Wet

Allergen Levels: _____
BM Pressure: _____

EXERCISE

- ☐ Heck yes, I worked out.
- ☐ I managed to exercise a bit.
- ☐ No, I haven't exercised at all.
- ☐ I did some stuff, and that counts.

DETAILS

FOOD / MEDICATION

Food / Drinks

Meds / Supplements	Time	Dose

☐ usual daily medication

Notes

I am grateful for...

M T W T F S S

DATE:

HOW ARE YOU *Feeling today?*

😍 Amazing!	🙂 Meh
😁 Great	😠 Not good
😊 Good	😣 Terrible!

RATE YOUR PAIN LEVEL

① ② ③ ④ ⑤ ⑥ ⑦ ⑧ ⑨ ⑩

WHAT ABOUT YOUR...?

Mood	① ② ③ ④ ⑤ ⑥ ⑦ ⑧ ⑨ ⑩
Energy Levels	① ② ③ ④ ⑤ ⑥ ⑦ ⑧ ⑨ ⑩
Mental Clarity	① ② ③ ④ ⑤ ⑥ ⑦ ⑧ ⑨ ⑩

PAIN & SYMPTOM DETAILS

	am	pm	front	back	other
	☐	☐			☐ Nausea
	☐	☐			☐ Diarrhea
	☐	☐			☐ Vomiting
	☐	☐			☐ Sore throat
	☐	☐			☐ Congestion
	☐	☐			☐ Coughing
	☐	☐			☐ Chills
	☐	☐			☐ Fever

SLEEP

hours _____

quality ① ② ③ ④ ⑤

STRESS LEVELS

None	Low	Medium	High	Max	@$#%!

WEATHER

☐ Cold ☐ Mild ☐ Hot
☐ Dry ☐ Humid ☐ Wet

Allergen Levels: _____
BM Pressure: _____

EXERCISE

☐ Heck yes, I worked out.
☐ I managed to exercise a bit.
☐ No, I haven't exercised at all.
☐ I did some stuff, and that counts.

DETAILS

FOOD / MEDICATION

Food / Drinks

Meds / Supplements	Time	Dose

☐ usual daily medication

Notes

_____

I am grateful for...

M T W T F S S   DATE:

HOW ARE YOU *Feeling today?*

😍 Amazing!	🙂 Meh
😁 Great	😠 Not good
😊 Good	😖 Terrible!

RATE YOUR PAIN LEVEL

① ② ③ ④ ⑤ ⑥ ⑦ ⑧ ⑨ ⑩

WHAT ABOUT YOUR...?

Mood	① ② ③ ④ ⑤ ⑥ ⑦ ⑧ ⑨ ⑩
Energy Levels	① ② ③ ④ ⑤ ⑥ ⑦ ⑧ ⑨ ⑩
Mental Clarity	① ② ③ ④ ⑤ ⑥ ⑦ ⑧ ⑨ ⑩

PAIN & SYMPTOM DETAILS

	am	pm	front	back	other
_____	☐	☐			☐ Nausea
_____	☐	☐			☐ Diarrhea
_____	☐	☐			☐ Vomiting
_____	☐	☐			☐ Sore throat
_____	☐	☐			☐ Congestion
_____	☐	☐			☐ Coughing
_____	☐	☐			☐ Chills
_____	☐	☐			☐ Fever

SLEEP

hours
_____

quality
① ② ③ ④ ⑤

STRESS LEVELS

None	Low	Medium	High	Max	@$#%!

WEATHER

☐ Cold ☐ Mild ☐ Hot
☐ Dry   ☐ Humid ☐ Wet

Allergen Levels: _____
BM Pressure: _____

EXERCISE

☐ Heck yes, I worked out.
☐ I managed to exercise a bit.
☐ No, I haven't exercised at all.
☐ I did some stuff, and that counts.

DETAILS

FOOD / MEDICATION

Food / Drinks

Meds / Supplements	Time	Dose

☐ usual daily medication

Notes

I am grateful for...

M T W T F S S   DATE:

HOW ARE YOU Feeling today?

😍 Amazing!	🙂 Meh
😁 Great	😠 Not good
😊 Good	😖 Terrible!

RATE YOUR PAIN LEVEL

① ② ③ ④ ⑤ ⑥ ⑦ ⑧ ⑨ ⑩

WHAT ABOUT YOUR...?

Mood	① ② ③ ④ ⑤ ⑥ ⑦ ⑧ ⑨ ⑩
Energy Levels	① ② ③ ④ ⑤ ⑥ ⑦ ⑧ ⑨ ⑩
Mental Clarity	① ② ③ ④ ⑤ ⑥ ⑦ ⑧ ⑨ ⑩

PAIN & SYMPTOM DETAILS

	am	pm	front	back	other
	☐	☐			☐ Nausea
	☐	☐			☐ Diarrhea
	☐	☐			☐ Vomiting
	☐	☐			☐ Sore throat
	☐	☐			☐ Congestion
	☐	☐			☐ Coughing
	☐	☐			☐ Chills
	☐	☐			☐ Fever

SLEEP

hours _____   *quality* ① ② ③ ④ ⑤

STRESS LEVELS

None	Low	Medium	High	Max	@$#%!

WEATHER

☐ Cold   ☐ Mild   ☐ Hot
☐ Dry   ☐ Humid   ☐ Wet
Allergen Levels: _____
BM Pressure: _____

EXERCISE

☐ Heck yes, I worked out.
☐ I managed to exercise a bit.
☐ No, I haven't exercised at all.
☐ I did some stuff, and that counts.

DETAILS

FOOD / MEDICATION

Food / Drinks

Meds / Supplements	Time	Dose

☐ usual daily medication

Notes

I am grateful for...

HOW ARE YOU *Feeling today?*

😍 Amazing!	🙂 Meh
😁 Great	😣 Not good
🙂 Good	😖 Terrible!

RATE YOUR PAIN LEVEL
① ② ③ ④ ⑤ ⑥ ⑦ ⑧ ⑨ ⑩

WHAT ABOUT YOUR...?

Mood	① ② ③ ④ ⑤ ⑥ ⑦ ⑧ ⑨ ⑩
Energy Levels	① ② ③ ④ ⑤ ⑥ ⑦ ⑧ ⑨ ⑩
Mental Clarity	① ② ③ ④ ⑤ ⑥ ⑦ ⑧ ⑨ ⑩

PAIN & SYMPTOM DETAILS

	am	pm	*front*	*back*	*other*
_____	☐	☐			☐ Nausea
_____	☐	☐			☐ Diarrhea
_____	☐	☐			☐ Vomiting
_____	☐	☐			☐ Sore throat
_____	☐	☐			☐ Congestion
_____	☐	☐			☐ Coughing
_____	☐	☐			☐ Chills
_____	☐	☐			☐ Fever

SLEEP

hours
_____

quality
① ② ③ ④ ⑤

STRESS LEVELS

None	Low	Medium	High	Max	@$#%!

WEATHER

☐ Cold ☐ Mild ☐ Hot
☐ Dry ☐ Humid ☐ Wet
Allergen Levels: _____
BM Pressure: _____

EXERCISE

☐ Heck yes, I worked out.
☐ I managed to exercise a bit.
☐ No, I haven't exercised at all.
☐ I did some stuff, and that counts.

DETAILS

FOOD / MEDICATION

Food / Drinks	Meds / Supplements	Time	Dose

☐ usual daily medication

Notes
_____
_____

I am grateful for...
_____

HOW ARE YOU *Feeling today?*

😍 Amazing!	🙂 Meh
😁 Great	😠 Not good
😊 Good	😵 Terrible!

RATE YOUR PAIN LEVEL

① ② ③ ④ ⑤ ⑥ ⑦ ⑧ ⑨ ⑩

WHAT ABOUT YOUR...?

Mood	① ② ③ ④ ⑤ ⑥ ⑦ ⑧ ⑨ ⑩
Energy Levels	① ② ③ ④ ⑤ ⑥ ⑦ ⑧ ⑨ ⑩
Mental Clarity	① ② ③ ④ ⑤ ⑥ ⑦ ⑧ ⑨ ⑩

PAIN & SYMPTOM DETAILS

	am	pm	front	back	other
_____	☐	☐			☐ Nausea
_____	☐	☐			☐ Diarrhea
_____	☐	☐			☐ Vomiting
_____	☐	☐			☐ Sore throat
_____	☐	☐			☐ Congestion
_____	☐	☐			☐ Coughing
_____	☐	☐			☐ Chills
_____	☐	☐			☐ Fever

SLEEP

hours _____

quality ① ② ③ ④ ⑤

STRESS LEVELS

None	Low	Medium	High	Max	@$#%!

WEATHER

☐ Cold   ☐ Mild   ☐ Hot
☐ Dry   ☐ Humid   ☐ Wet

Allergen Levels: _____

BM Pressure: _____

EXERCISE

☐ Heck yes, I worked out.
☐ I managed to exercise a bit.
☐ No, I haven't exercised at all.
☐ I did some stuff, and that counts.

DETAILS

FOOD / MEDICATION

Food / Drinks

Meds / Supplements	Time	Dose

☐ usual daily medication

Notes
_____
_____

I am grateful for...

HOW ARE YOU *Feeling today?*

Amazing!	Meh
Great	Not good
Good	Terrible!

RATE YOUR PAIN LEVEL

① ② ③ ④ ⑤ ⑥ ⑦ ⑧ ⑨ ⑩

WHAT ABOUT YOUR...?

Mood	① ② ③ ④ ⑤ ⑥ ⑦ ⑧ ⑨ ⑩
Energy Levels	① ② ③ ④ ⑤ ⑥ ⑦ ⑧ ⑨ ⑩
Mental Clarity	① ② ③ ④ ⑤ ⑥ ⑦ ⑧ ⑨ ⑩

PAIN & SYMPTOM DETAILS

	am	pm	*front*	*back*	*other*
	☐	☐			☐ Nausea
	☐	☐			☐ Diarrhea
	☐	☐			☐ Vomiting
	☐	☐			☐ Sore throat
	☐	☐			☐ Congestion
	☐	☐			☐ Coughing
	☐	☐			☐ Chills
	☐	☐			☐ Fever

SLEEP

hours _____   *quality* ① ② ③ ④ ⑤

STRESS LEVELS

None	Low	Medium	High	Max	@$#%!

WEATHER

☐ Cold   ☐ Mild   ☐ Hot
☐ Dry   ☐ Humid   ☐ Wet
Allergen Levels: _____
BM Pressure: _____

EXERCISE

☐ Heck yes, I worked out.
☐ I managed to exercise a bit.
☐ No, I haven't exercised at all.
☐ I did some stuff, and that counts.

DETAILS

FOOD / MEDICATION

Food / Drinks

Meds / Supplements	Time	Dose

☐ usual daily medication

Notes

I am grateful for…

M T W T F S S   DATE:

HOW ARE YOU *Feeling today?*

😍 Amazing!	🙂 Meh
😁 Great	😣 Not good
🙂 Good	😖 Terrible!

RATE YOUR PAIN LEVEL

① ② ③ ④ ⑤ ⑥ ⑦ ⑧ ⑨ ⑩

WHAT ABOUT YOUR...?

Mood	① ② ③ ④ ⑤ ⑥ ⑦ ⑧ ⑨ ⑩
Energy Levels	① ② ③ ④ ⑤ ⑥ ⑦ ⑧ ⑨ ⑩
Mental Clarity	① ② ③ ④ ⑤ ⑥ ⑦ ⑧ ⑨ ⑩

PAIN & SYMPTOM DETAILS

	am	pm	*front*	*back*	*other*
_____	☐	☐			☐ Nausea
_____	☐	☐			☐ Diarrhea
_____	☐	☐			☐ Vomiting
_____	☐	☐			☐ Sore throat
_____	☐	☐			☐ Congestion
_____	☐	☐			☐ Coughing
_____	☐	☐			☐ Chills
_____	☐	☐			☐ Fever

SLEEP

hours
_____

quality
① ② ③ ④ ⑤

STRESS LEVELS

None	Low	Medium	High	Max	@$#%!

WEATHER

☐ Cold   ☐ Mild   ☐ Hot
☐ Dry   ☐ Humid   ☐ Wet
Allergen Levels: _____
BM Pressure: _____

EXERCISE

☐ Heck yes, I worked out.
☐ I managed to exercise a bit.
☐ No, I haven't exercised at all.
☐ I did some stuff, and that counts.

DETAILS

FOOD / MEDICATION

Food / Drinks	Meds / Supplements	Time	Dose

☐ usual daily medication

Notes

I am grateful for...

HOW ARE YOU *Feeling today?*

Amazing!	Meh
Great	Not good
Good	Terrible!

RATE YOUR PAIN LEVEL

①②③④⑤⑥⑦⑧⑨⑩

WHAT ABOUT YOUR...?

Mood	①②③④⑤⑥⑦⑧⑨⑩
Energy Levels	①②③④⑤⑥⑦⑧⑨⑩
Mental Clarity	①②③④⑤⑥⑦⑧⑨⑩

PAIN & SYMPTOM DETAILS

	am	pm
_____	☐	☐
_____	☐	☐
_____	☐	☐
_____	☐	☐
_____	☐	☐
_____	☐	☐
_____	☐	☐
_____	☐	☐

front   *back*

other

- ☐ Nausea
- ☐ Diarrhea
- ☐ Vomiting
- ☐ Sore throat
- ☐ Congestion
- ☐ Coughing
- ☐ Chills
- ☐ Fever

SLEEP

hours
_____

quality
①②③④⑤

STRESS LEVELS

None	Low	Medium	High	Max	@$#%!

WEATHER

- ☐ Cold
- ☐ Dry
- ☐ Mild
- ☐ Humid
- ☐ Hot
- ☐ Wet

Allergen Levels: _____

BM Pressure: _____

EXERCISE

- ☐ Heck yes, I worked out.
- ☐ I managed to exercise a bit.
- ☐ No, I haven't exercised at all.
- ☐ I did some stuff, and that counts.

DETAILS

FOOD / MEDICATION

Food / Drinks

Meds / Supplements	Time	Dose

☐ usual daily medication

Notes
_____

I am grateful for...

HOW ARE YOU *Feeling today?*

Amazing!	Meh
Great	Not good
Good	Terrible!

RATE YOUR PAIN LEVEL

① ② ③ ④ ⑤ ⑥ ⑦ ⑧ ⑨ ⑩

WHAT ABOUT YOUR...?

Mood	① ② ③ ④ ⑤ ⑥ ⑦ ⑧ ⑨ ⑩
Energy Levels	① ② ③ ④ ⑤ ⑥ ⑦ ⑧ ⑨ ⑩
Mental Clarity	① ② ③ ④ ⑤ ⑥ ⑦ ⑧ ⑨ ⑩

PAIN & SYMPTOM DETAILS

	am	pm		front	back	other
	☐	☐				☐ Nausea
	☐	☐				☐ Diarrhea
	☐	☐				☐ Vomiting
	☐	☐				☐ Sore throat
	☐	☐				☐ Congestion
	☐	☐				☐ Coughing
	☐	☐				☐ Chills
	☐	☐				☐ Fever

SLEEP

hours _____ *quality* ① ② ③ ④ ⑤

STRESS LEVELS

None	Low	Medium	High	Max	@$#%!

WEATHER

☐ Cold ☐ Mild ☐ Hot
☐ Dry ☐ Humid ☐ Wet
Allergen Levels: _____
BM Pressure: _____

EXERCISE

☐ Heck yes, I worked out.
☐ I managed to exercise a bit.
☐ No, I haven't exercised at all.
☐ I did some stuff, and that counts.

DETAILS

FOOD / MEDICATION

Food / Drinks

Meds / Supplements	Time	Dose

☐ usual daily medication

Notes

I am grateful for…

HOW ARE YOU *Feeling today?*

☺ Amazing!	☺ Meh
☺ Great	☹ Not good
☺ Good	☹ Terrible!

RATE YOUR PAIN LEVEL

① ② ③ ④ ⑤ ⑥ ⑦ ⑧ ⑨ ⑩

WHAT ABOUT YOUR...?

Mood	① ② ③ ④ ⑤ ⑥ ⑦ ⑧ ⑨ ⑩
Energy Levels	① ② ③ ④ ⑤ ⑥ ⑦ ⑧ ⑨ ⑩
Mental Clarity	① ② ③ ④ ⑤ ⑥ ⑦ ⑧ ⑨ ⑩

PAIN & SYMPTOM DETAILS

	am	pm	front	back	other
	☐	☐			☐ Nausea
	☐	☐			☐ Diarrhea
	☐	☐			☐ Vomiting
	☐	☐			☐ Sore throat
	☐	☐			☐ Congestion
	☐	☐			☐ Coughing
	☐	☐			☐ Chills
	☐	☐			☐ Fever

SLEEP

hours _____

quality ① ② ③ ④ ⑤

STRESS LEVELS

None	Low	Medium	High	Max	@$#%!

WEATHER

☐ Cold   ☐ Mild   ☐ Hot
☐ Dry   ☐ Humid   ☐ Wet

Allergen Levels: _____
BM Pressure: _____

EXERCISE

☐ Heck yes, I worked out.
☐ I managed to exercise a bit.
☐ No, I haven't exercised at all.
☐ I did some stuff, and that counts.

DETAILS

FOOD / MEDICATION

Food / Drinks

Meds / Supplements	Time	Dose

☐ usual daily medication

Notes
_____
_____

I am grateful for...

M T W T F S S   DATE:

HOW ARE YOU Feeling today?

Amazing!	Meh
Great	Not good
Good	Terrible!

RATE YOUR PAIN LEVEL

① ② ③ ④ ⑤ ⑥ ⑦ ⑧ ⑨ ⑩

WHAT ABOUT YOUR...?

Mood	①	②	③	④	⑤	⑥	⑦	⑧	⑨	⑩
Energy Levels	①	②	③	④	⑤	⑥	⑦	⑧	⑨	⑩
Mental Clarity	①	②	③	④	⑤	⑥	⑦	⑧	⑨	⑩

PAIN & SYMPTOM DETAILS

	am	pm
_____	☐	☐
_____	☐	☐
_____	☐	☐
_____	☐	☐
_____	☐	☐
_____	☐	☐
_____	☐	☐
_____	☐	☐

front   *back*

other

☐ Nausea
☐ Diarrhea
☐ Vomiting
☐ Sore throat
☐ Congestion
☐ Coughing
☐ Chills
☐ Fever

SLEEP

hours
_____

quality
① ② ③ ④ ⑤

STRESS LEVELS

None	Low	Medium	High	Max	@$#%!

WEATHER

☐ Cold   ☐ Mild   ☐ Hot
☐ Dry   ☐ Humid   ☐ Wet

Allergen Levels: _____
BM Pressure: _____

EXERCISE

☐ Heck yes, I worked out.
☐ I managed to exercise a bit.
☐ No, I haven't exercised at all.
☐ I did some stuff, and that counts.

DETAILS

FOOD / MEDICATION

Food / Drinks

Meds / Supplements	Time	Dose

☐ usual daily medication

Notes
_____
_____

I am grateful for...

HOW ARE YOU Feeling today?

😍 Amazing!	🙂 Meh
😁 Great	😣 Not good
😊 Good	😖 Terrible!

RATE YOUR PAIN LEVEL

① ② ③ ④ ⑤ ⑥ ⑦ ⑧ ⑨ ⑩

WHAT ABOUT YOUR...?

Mood	① ② ③ ④ ⑤ ⑥ ⑦ ⑧ ⑨ ⑩
Energy Levels	① ② ③ ④ ⑤ ⑥ ⑦ ⑧ ⑨ ⑩
Mental Clarity	① ② ③ ④ ⑤ ⑥ ⑦ ⑧ ⑨ ⑩

PAIN & SYMPTOM DETAILS

	am	pm	front	back	other
	☐	☐			☐ Nausea
	☐	☐			☐ Diarrhea
	☐	☐			☐ Vomiting
	☐	☐			☐ Sore throat
	☐	☐			☐ Congestion
	☐	☐			☐ Coughing
	☐	☐			☐ Chills
	☐	☐			☐ Fever

SLEEP

hours
_____

quality
① ② ③ ④ ⑤

STRESS LEVELS

None	Low	Medium	High	Max	@$#%!

WEATHER

☐ Cold   ☐ Mild   ☐ Hot
☐ Dry   ☐ Humid   ☐ Wet
Allergen Levels: _____
BM Pressure: _____

EXERCISE

☐ Heck yes, I worked out.
☐ I managed to exercise a bit.
☐ No, I haven't exercised at all.
☐ I did some stuff, and that counts.

DETAILS

FOOD / MEDICATION

Food / Drinks

Meds / Supplements	Time	Dose

☐ usual daily medication

Notes

I am grateful for...

M T W T F S S

DATE:

HOW ARE YOU *Feeling today?*

Amazing!	Meh
Great	Not good
Good	Terrible!

RATE YOUR PAIN LEVEL

① ② ③ ④ ⑤ ⑥ ⑦ ⑧ ⑨ ⑩

WHAT ABOUT YOUR...?

Mood	① ② ③ ④ ⑤ ⑥ ⑦ ⑧ ⑨ ⑩
Energy Levels	① ② ③ ④ ⑤ ⑥ ⑦ ⑧ ⑨ ⑩
Mental Clarity	① ② ③ ④ ⑤ ⑥ ⑦ ⑧ ⑨ ⑩

PAIN & SYMPTOM DETAILS

	am	pm	front	back	other
	☐	☐			☐ Nausea
	☐	☐			☐ Diarrhea
	☐	☐			☐ Vomiting
	☐	☐			☐ Sore throat
	☐	☐			☐ Congestion
	☐	☐			☐ Coughing
	☐	☐			☐ Chills
	☐	☐			☐ Fever

SLEEP

hours _____

quality ① ② ③ ④ ⑤

STRESS LEVELS

None	Low	Medium	High	Max	@$#%!

WEATHER

☐ Cold ☐ Mild ☐ Hot
☐ Dry ☐ Humid ☐ Wet

Allergen Levels: _____
BM Pressure: _____

EXERCISE

☐ Heck yes, I worked out.
☐ I managed to exercise a bit.
☐ No, I haven't exercised at all.
☐ I did some stuff, and that counts.

DETAILS

FOOD / MEDICATION

Food / Drinks

Meds / Supplements	Time	Dose

☐ usual daily medication

Notes

I am grateful for...

HOW ARE YOU Feeling today?

Amazing!	Meh
Great	Not good
Good	Terrible!

RATE YOUR PAIN LEVEL

① ② ③ ④ ⑤ ⑥ ⑦ ⑧ ⑨ ⑩

WHAT ABOUT YOUR...?

Mood	① ② ③ ④ ⑤ ⑥ ⑦ ⑧ ⑨ ⑩
Energy Levels	① ② ③ ④ ⑤ ⑥ ⑦ ⑧ ⑨ ⑩
Mental Clarity	① ② ③ ④ ⑤ ⑥ ⑦ ⑧ ⑨ ⑩

PAIN & SYMPTOM DETAILS

	am	pm	front	back	other
	☐	☐			☐ Nausea
	☐	☐			☐ Diarrhea
	☐	☐			☐ Vomiting
	☐	☐			☐ Sore throat
	☐	☐			☐ Congestion
	☐	☐			☐ Coughing
	☐	☐			☐ Chills
	☐	☐			☐ Fever

SLEEP

hours _____   quality ① ② ③ ④ ⑤

STRESS LEVELS

None	Low	Medium	High	Max	@$#%!

WEATHER

☐ Cold   ☐ Mild   ☐ Hot
☐ Dry   ☐ Humid   ☐ Wet

Allergen Levels: _____
BM Pressure: _____

EXERCISE

☐ Heck yes, I worked out.
☐ I managed to exercise a bit.
☐ No, I haven't exercised at all.
☐ I did some stuff, and that counts.

DETAILS

FOOD / MEDICATION

Food / Drinks

Meds / Supplements	Time	Dose

☐ usual daily medication

Notes

I am grateful for...

HOW ARE YOU *Feeling today?*

😍 Amazing!	🙂 Meh
😁 Great	😣 Not good
😊 Good	😖 Terrible!

RATE YOUR PAIN LEVEL

① ② ③ ④ ⑤ ⑥ ⑦ ⑧ ⑨ ⑩

WHAT ABOUT YOUR...?

Mood	① ② ③ ④ ⑤ ⑥ ⑦ ⑧ ⑨ ⑩
Energy Levels	① ② ③ ④ ⑤ ⑥ ⑦ ⑧ ⑨ ⑩
Mental Clarity	① ② ③ ④ ⑤ ⑥ ⑦ ⑧ ⑨ ⑩

PAIN & SYMPTOM DETAILS

	am	pm	*front*	*back*	*other*
_____	☐	☐			☐ Nausea
_____	☐	☐			☐ Diarrhea
_____	☐	☐			☐ Vomiting
_____	☐	☐			☐ Sore throat
_____	☐	☐			☐ Congestion
_____	☐	☐			☐ Coughing
_____	☐	☐			☐ Chills
_____	☐	☐			☐ Fever

SLEEP

hours   *quality*
_____   ① ② ③ ④ ⑤

STRESS LEVELS

None	Low	Medium	High	Max	@$#%!

WEATHER

☐ Cold   ☐ Mild   ☐ Hot
☐ Dry   ☐ Humid   ☐ Wet
Allergen Levels: _____
BM Pressure: _____

EXERCISE

☐ Heck yes, I worked out.
☐ I managed to exercise a bit.
☐ No, I haven't exercised at all.
☐ I did some stuff, and that counts.

DETAILS

FOOD / MEDICATION

Food / Drinks	Meds / Supplements	Time	Dose

☐ usual daily medication

Notes
_____
_____

I am grateful for...
_____

M T W T F S S   DATE:

HOW ARE YOU *Feeling today?*

😍 Amazing!	🙂 Meh
😁 Great	😠 Not good
🙂 Good	😣 Terrible!

RATE YOUR PAIN LEVEL

① ② ③ ④ ⑤ ⑥ ⑦ ⑧ ⑨ ⑩

WHAT ABOUT YOUR...?

Mood	① ② ③ ④ ⑤ ⑥ ⑦ ⑧ ⑨ ⑩
Energy Levels	① ② ③ ④ ⑤ ⑥ ⑦ ⑧ ⑨ ⑩
Mental Clarity	① ② ③ ④ ⑤ ⑥ ⑦ ⑧ ⑨ ⑩

PAIN & SYMPTOM DETAILS

	am	pm	*front*	*back*	*other*
_____	☐	☐			☐ Nausea
_____	☐	☐			☐ Diarrhea
_____	☐	☐			☐ Vomiting
_____	☐	☐			☐ Sore throat
_____	☐	☐			☐ Congestion
_____	☐	☐			☐ Coughing
_____	☐	☐			☐ Chills
_____	☐	☐			☐ Fever

SLEEP

hours _____   *quality* ① ② ③ ④ ⑤

STRESS LEVELS

None	Low	Medium	High	Max	@$#%!

WEATHER

☐ Cold   ☐ Mild   ☐ Hot
☐ Dry   ☐ Humid ☐ Wet
Allergen Levels: _____
BM Pressure: _____

EXERCISE

☐ Heck yes, I worked out.
☐ I managed to exercise a bit.
☐ No, I haven't exercised at all.
☐ I did some stuff, and that counts.

DETAILS

FOOD / MEDICATION

Food / Drinks

Meds / Supplements	Time	Dose

☐ usual daily medication

Notes
_____
_____

I am grateful for...

HOW ARE YOU *Feeling today?*

😍 Amazing!	🙂 Meh
😁 Great	😠 Not good
😊 Good	😖 Terrible!

RATE YOUR PAIN LEVEL

① ② ③ ④ ⑤ ⑥ ⑦ ⑧ ⑨ ⑩

WHAT ABOUT YOUR...?

Mood	① ② ③ ④ ⑤ ⑥ ⑦ ⑧ ⑨ ⑩
Energy Levels	① ② ③ ④ ⑤ ⑥ ⑦ ⑧ ⑨ ⑩
Mental Clarity	① ② ③ ④ ⑤ ⑥ ⑦ ⑧ ⑨ ⑩

PAIN & SYMPTOM DETAILS

	am	pm	front	back	other
	☐	☐			☐ Nausea
	☐	☐			☐ Diarrhea
	☐	☐			☐ Vomiting
	☐	☐			☐ Sore throat
	☐	☐			☐ Congestion
	☐	☐			☐ Coughing
	☐	☐			☐ Chills
	☐	☐			☐ Fever

SLEEP

hours _____   *quality* ① ② ③ ④ ⑤

STRESS LEVELS

None	Low	Medium	High	Max	@$#%!

WEATHER

☐ Cold   ☐ Mild   ☐ Hot
☐ Dry   ☐ Humid   ☐ Wet
Allergen Levels: _____
BM Pressure: _____

EXERCISE

☐ Heck yes, I worked out.
☐ I managed to exercise a bit.
☐ No, I haven't exercised at all.
☐ I did some stuff, and that counts.

DETAILS

FOOD / MEDICATION

Food / Drinks	Meds / Supplements	Time	Dose

☐ usual daily medication

Notes _____
_____

I am grateful for...

M T W T F S S   DATE:

HOW ARE YOU Feeling today?

Amazing!	Meh
Great	Not good
Good	Terrible!

RATE YOUR PAIN LEVEL

① ② ③ ④ ⑤ ⑥ ⑦ ⑧ ⑨ ⑩

WHAT ABOUT YOUR...?

Mood	① ② ③ ④ ⑤ ⑥ ⑦ ⑧ ⑨ ⑩
Energy Levels	① ② ③ ④ ⑤ ⑥ ⑦ ⑧ ⑨ ⑩
Mental Clarity	① ② ③ ④ ⑤ ⑥ ⑦ ⑧ ⑨ ⑩

PAIN & SYMPTOM DETAILS

	am	pm	front	back	other
	☐	☐			☐ Nausea
	☐	☐			☐ Diarrhea
	☐	☐			☐ Vomiting
	☐	☐			☐ Sore throat
	☐	☐			☐ Congestion
	☐	☐			☐ Coughing
	☐	☐			☐ Chills
	☐	☐			☐ Fever

SLEEP

hours _____

quality ① ② ③ ④ ⑤

STRESS LEVELS

None	Low	Medium	High	Max	@$#%!

WEATHER

☐ Cold   ☐ Mild   ☐ Hot
☐ Dry   ☐ Humid   ☐ Wet
Allergen Levels: _____
BM Pressure: _____

EXERCISE

☐ Heck yes, I worked out.
☐ I managed to exercise a bit.
☐ No, I haven't exercised at all.
☐ I did some stuff, and that counts.

DETAILS

FOOD / MEDICATION

Food / Drinks

Meds / Supplements	Time	Dose

☐ usual daily medication

Notes

I am grateful for...

M T W T F S S

DATE:

HOW ARE YOU *Feeling today?*

Amazing!	Meh
Great	Not good
Good	Terrible!

RATE YOUR PAIN LEVEL

① ② ③ ④ ⑤ ⑥ ⑦ ⑧ ⑨ ⑩

WHAT ABOUT YOUR...?

Mood	① ② ③ ④ ⑤ ⑥ ⑦ ⑧ ⑨ ⑩
Energy Levels	① ② ③ ④ ⑤ ⑥ ⑦ ⑧ ⑨ ⑩
Mental Clarity	① ② ③ ④ ⑤ ⑥ ⑦ ⑧ ⑨ ⑩

PAIN & SYMPTOM DETAILS

	am	pm	front	back	other
_____	☐	☐			☐ Nausea
_____	☐	☐			☐ Diarrhea
_____	☐	☐			☐ Vomiting
_____	☐	☐			☐ Sore throat
_____	☐	☐			☐ Congestion
_____	☐	☐			☐ Coughing
_____	☐	☐			☐ Chills
_____	☐	☐			☐ Fever

SLEEP

hours
_____

quality
① ② ③ ④ ⑤

STRESS LEVELS

None	Low	Medium	High	Max	@$#%!

WEATHER

☐ Cold ☐ Mild ☐ Hot
☐ Dry ☐ Humid ☐ Wet

Allergen Levels: _____
BM Pressure: _____

EXERCISE

☐ Heck yes, I worked out.
☐ I managed to exercise a bit.
☐ No, I haven't exercised at all.
☐ I did some stuff, and that counts.

DETAILS

FOOD / MEDICATION

Food / Drinks

Meds / Supplements	Time	Dose

☐ usual daily medication

Notes
_____

I am grateful for...

M T W T F S S   DATE:

HOW ARE YOU *Feeling today?*

Amazing!	Meh
Great	Not good
Good	Terrible!

RATE YOUR PAIN LEVEL

① ② ③ ④ ⑤ ⑥ ⑦ ⑧ ⑨ ⑩

WHAT ABOUT YOUR...?

Mood	① ② ③ ④ ⑤ ⑥ ⑦ ⑧ ⑨ ⑩
Energy Levels	① ② ③ ④ ⑤ ⑥ ⑦ ⑧ ⑨ ⑩
Mental Clarity	① ② ③ ④ ⑤ ⑥ ⑦ ⑧ ⑨ ⑩

PAIN & SYMPTOM DETAILS

	am	pm	*front*	*back*	*other*
_____	☐	☐			☐ Nausea
_____	☐	☐			☐ Diarrhea
_____	☐	☐			☐ Vomiting
_____	☐	☐			☐ Sore throat
_____	☐	☐			☐ Congestion
_____	☐	☐			☐ Coughing
_____	☐	☐			☐ Chills
_____	☐	☐			☐ Fever

SLEEP

hours
_____

quality
① ② ③ ④ ⑤

STRESS LEVELS

None	Low	Medium	High	Max	@$#%!

WEATHER

☐ Cold   ☐ Mild   ☐ Hot
☐ Dry   ☐ Humid   ☐ Wet
Allergen Levels: _____
BM Pressure: _____

EXERCISE

☐ Heck yes, I worked out.
☐ I managed to exercise a bit.
☐ No, I haven't exercised at all.
☐ I did some stuff, and that counts.

DETAILS

FOOD / MEDICATION

Food / Drinks

Meds / Supplements	Time	Dose

☐ usual daily medication

Notes
_____

I am grateful for...

HOW ARE YOU *Feeling today?*

😍 Amazing!	🙂 Meh
😁 Great	😣 Not good
😊 Good	😖 Terrible!

RATE YOUR PAIN LEVEL

① ② ③ ④ ⑤ ⑥ ⑦ ⑧ ⑨ ⑩

WHAT ABOUT YOUR...?

Mood	① ② ③ ④ ⑤ ⑥ ⑦ ⑧ ⑨ ⑩
Energy Levels	① ② ③ ④ ⑤ ⑥ ⑦ ⑧ ⑨ ⑩
Mental Clarity	① ② ③ ④ ⑤ ⑥ ⑦ ⑧ ⑨ ⑩

PAIN & SYMPTOM DETAILS

	am	pm	*front*	*back*	*other*
_____	☐	☐			☐ Nausea
_____	☐	☐			☐ Diarrhea
_____	☐	☐			☐ Vomiting
_____	☐	☐			☐ Sore throat
_____	☐	☐			☐ Congestion
_____	☐	☐			☐ Coughing
_____	☐	☐			☐ Chills
_____	☐	☐			☐ Fever

SLEEP

hours
_____

quality
① ② ③ ④ ⑤

STRESS LEVELS

None	Low	Medium	High	Max	@$#%!

WEATHER

☐ Cold ☐ Mild ☐ Hot
☐ Dry ☐ Humid ☐ Wet

Allergen Levels: _____
BM Pressure: _____

EXERCISE

☐ Heck yes, I worked out.
☐ I managed to exercise a bit.
☐ No, I haven't exercised at all.
☐ I did some stuff, and that counts.

DETAILS

FOOD / MEDICATION

Food / Drinks

Meds / Supplements	Time	Dose

☐ usual daily medication

Notes
_____
_____

I am grateful for...

M T W T F S S   DATE:

HOW ARE YOU Feeling today?

Amazing!	Meh
Great	Not good
Good	Terrible!

RATE YOUR PAIN LEVEL

① ② ③ ④ ⑤ ⑥ ⑦ ⑧ ⑨ ⑩

WHAT ABOUT YOUR...?

Mood	① ② ③ ④ ⑤ ⑥ ⑦ ⑧ ⑨ ⑩
Energy Levels	① ② ③ ④ ⑤ ⑥ ⑦ ⑧ ⑨ ⑩
Mental Clarity	① ② ③ ④ ⑤ ⑥ ⑦ ⑧ ⑨ ⑩

PAIN & SYMPTOM DETAILS

	am	pm	front	back	other
_____	☐	☐			☐ Nausea
_____	☐	☐			☐ Diarrhea
_____	☐	☐			☐ Vomiting
_____	☐	☐			☐ Sore throat
_____	☐	☐			☐ Congestion
_____	☐	☐			☐ Coughing
_____	☐	☐			☐ Chills
_____	☐	☐			☐ Fever

SLEEP

hours _____   quality ① ② ③ ④ ⑤

STRESS LEVELS

None	Low	Medium	High	Max	@$#%!

WEATHER

☐ Cold   ☐ Mild   ☐ Hot
☐ Dry   ☐ Humid   ☐ Wet
Allergen Levels: _____
BM Pressure: _____

EXERCISE

☐ Heck yes, I worked out.
☐ I managed to exercise a bit.
☐ No, I haven't exercised at all.
☐ I did some stuff, and that counts.

DETAILS

FOOD / MEDICATION

Food / Drinks

Meds / Supplements	Time	Dose

☐ usual daily medication

Notes

_____

I am grateful for...

HOW ARE YOU Feeling today?

Amazing!	Meh
Great	Not good
Good	Terrible!

RATE YOUR PAIN LEVEL

① ② ③ ④ ⑤ ⑥ ⑦ ⑧ ⑨ ⑩

WHAT ABOUT YOUR...?

Mood	① ② ③ ④ ⑤ ⑥ ⑦ ⑧ ⑨ ⑩
Energy Levels	① ② ③ ④ ⑤ ⑥ ⑦ ⑧ ⑨ ⑩
Mental Clarity	① ② ③ ④ ⑤ ⑥ ⑦ ⑧ ⑨ ⑩

PAIN & SYMPTOM DETAILS

	am	pm	front	back	other
	☐	☐			☐ Nausea
	☐	☐			☐ Diarrhea
	☐	☐			☐ Vomiting
	☐	☐			☐ Sore throat
	☐	☐			☐ Congestion
	☐	☐			☐ Coughing
	☐	☐			☐ Chills
	☐	☐			☐ Fever

SLEEP

hours _____   *quality* ① ② ③ ④ ⑤

STRESS LEVELS

None	Low	Medium	High	Max	@$#%!

WEATHER

☐ Cold   ☐ Mild   ☐ Hot
☐ Dry   ☐ Humid   ☐ Wet
Allergen Levels: _____
BM Pressure: _____

EXERCISE

☐ Heck yes, I worked out.
☐ I managed to exercise a bit.
☐ No, I haven't exercised at all.
☐ I did some stuff, and that counts.

DETAILS

FOOD / MEDICATION

Food / Drinks

Meds / Supplements	Time	Dose

☐ usual daily medication

Notes
_____
_____

I am grateful for...

HOW ARE YOU *Feeling today?*

😍 Amazing!	🙂 Meh
😁 Great	😠 Not good
😊 Good	😫 Terrible!

RATE YOUR PAIN LEVEL
① ② ③ ④ ⑤ ⑥ ⑦ ⑧ ⑨ ⑩

WHAT ABOUT YOUR...?

Mood	① ② ③ ④ ⑤ ⑥ ⑦ ⑧ ⑨ ⑩
Energy Levels	① ② ③ ④ ⑤ ⑥ ⑦ ⑧ ⑨ ⑩
Mental Clarity	① ② ③ ④ ⑤ ⑥ ⑦ ⑧ ⑨ ⑩

PAIN & SYMPTOM DETAILS

	am	pm
	☐	☐
	☐	☐
	☐	☐
	☐	☐
	☐	☐
	☐	☐
	☐	☐

front   *back*

other
- ☐ Nausea
- ☐ Diarrhea
- ☐ Vomiting
- ☐ Sore throat
- ☐ Congestion
- ☐ Coughing
- ☐ Chills
- ☐ Fever

SLEEP

hours _____

quality ① ② ③ ④ ⑤

STRESS LEVELS

None	Low	Medium	High	Max	@$#%!

WEATHER

☐ Cold   ☐ Mild   ☐ Hot
☐ Dry   ☐ Humid   ☐ Wet

Allergen Levels: _____
BM Pressure: _____

EXERCISE

☐ Heck yes, I worked out.
☐ I managed to exercise a bit.
☐ No, I haven't exercised at all.
☐ I did some stuff, and that counts.

DETAILS

FOOD / MEDICATION

Food / Drinks

Meds / Supplements	Time	Dose

☐ usual daily medication

Notes
_____

I am grateful for...

M T W T F S S

DATE:

HOW ARE YOU *Feeling today?*

😍 Amazing!	🙂 Meh
😁 Great	😠 Not good
🙂 Good	😖 Terrible!

RATE YOUR PAIN LEVEL

① ② ③ ④ ⑤ ⑥ ⑦ ⑧ ⑨ ⑩

WHAT ABOUT YOUR...?

Mood	① ② ③ ④ ⑤ ⑥ ⑦ ⑧ ⑨ ⑩
Energy Levels	① ② ③ ④ ⑤ ⑥ ⑦ ⑧ ⑨ ⑩
Mental Clarity	① ② ③ ④ ⑤ ⑥ ⑦ ⑧ ⑨ ⑩

PAIN & SYMPTOM DETAILS

	am	pm	front	back	other
	☐	☐			☐ Nausea
	☐	☐			☐ Diarrhea
	☐	☐			☐ Vomiting
	☐	☐			☐ Sore throat
	☐	☐			☐ Congestion
	☐	☐			☐ Coughing
	☐	☐			☐ Chills
	☐	☐			☐ Fever

SLEEP

hours
_____

quality
① ② ③ ④ ⑤

STRESS LEVELS

None	Low	Medium	High	Max	@$#%!

WEATHER

☐ Cold ☐ Mild ☐ Hot
☐ Dry ☐ Humid ☐ Wet

Allergen Levels: _____
BM Pressure: _____

EXERCISE

☐ Heck yes, I worked out.
☐ I managed to exercise a bit.
☐ No, I haven't exercised at all.
☐ I did some stuff, and that counts.

DETAILS

FOOD / MEDICATION

Food / Drinks

Meds / Supplements	Time	Dose

☐ usual daily medication

Notes
_____
_____

I am grateful for...

HOW ARE YOU *Feeling today?*

😍 Amazing!	🙂 Meh
😁 Great	😠 Not good
🙂 Good	😤 Terrible!

RATE YOUR PAIN LEVEL

① ② ③ ④ ⑤ ⑥ ⑦ ⑧ ⑨ ⑩

WHAT ABOUT YOUR...?

Mood	① ② ③ ④ ⑤ ⑥ ⑦ ⑧ ⑨ ⑩
Energy Levels	① ② ③ ④ ⑤ ⑥ ⑦ ⑧ ⑨ ⑩
Mental Clarity	① ② ③ ④ ⑤ ⑥ ⑦ ⑧ ⑨ ⑩

PAIN & SYMPTOM DETAILS

	am	pm	front	back	other
_____	☐	☐			☐ Nausea
_____	☐	☐			☐ Diarrhea
_____	☐	☐			☐ Vomiting
_____	☐	☐			☐ Sore throat
_____	☐	☐			☐ Congestion
_____	☐	☐			☐ Coughing
_____	☐	☐			☐ Chills
_____	☐	☐			☐ Fever

SLEEP

hours
_____

quality
① ② ③ ④ ⑤

STRESS LEVELS

None	Low	Medium	High	Max	@$#%!

WEATHER

☐ Cold   ☐ Mild   ☐ Hot
☐ Dry   ☐ Humid   ☐ Wet
Allergen Levels: _____
BM Pressure: _____

EXERCISE

☐ Heck yes, I worked out.
☐ I managed to exercise a bit.
☐ No, I haven't exercised at all.
☐ I did some stuff, and that counts.

DETAILS

FOOD / MEDICATION

Food / Drinks

Meds / Supplements	Time	Dose

☐ usual daily medication

Notes
_____

I am grateful for...

M T W T F S S

DATE:

HOW ARE YOU Feeling today?

Amazing!	Meh
Great	Not good
Good	Terrible!

RATE YOUR PAIN LEVEL

① ② ③ ④ ⑤ ⑥ ⑦ ⑧ ⑨ ⑩

WHAT ABOUT YOUR...?

Mood	① ② ③ ④ ⑤ ⑥ ⑦ ⑧ ⑨ ⑩
Energy Levels	① ② ③ ④ ⑤ ⑥ ⑦ ⑧ ⑨ ⑩
Mental Clarity	① ② ③ ④ ⑤ ⑥ ⑦ ⑧ ⑨ ⑩

PAIN & SYMPTOM DETAILS

	am	pm	front	back	other
	☐	☐			☐ Nausea
	☐	☐			☐ Diarrhea
	☐	☐			☐ Vomiting
	☐	☐			☐ Sore throat
	☐	☐			☐ Congestion
	☐	☐			☐ Coughing
	☐	☐			☐ Chills
	☐	☐			☐ Fever

SLEEP

hours
_____

quality
① ② ③ ④ ⑤

STRESS LEVELS

None	Low	Medium	High	Max	@$#%!

WEATHER

☐ Cold   ☐ Mild   ☐ Hot
☐ Dry   ☐ Humid   ☐ Wet
Allergen Levels: _____
BM Pressure: _____

EXERCISE

☐ Heck yes, I worked out.
☐ I managed to exercise a bit.
☐ No, I haven't exercised at all.
☐ I did some stuff, and that counts.

DETAILS

FOOD / MEDICATION

Food / Drinks

Meds / Supplements	Time	Dose

☐ usual daily medication

Notes

I am grateful for…

HOW ARE YOU *Feeling today?*

😍 Amazing!	🙂 Meh
😁 Great	😠 Not good
🙂 Good	😣 Terrible!

RATE YOUR PAIN LEVEL

①②③④⑤⑥⑦⑧⑨⑩

WHAT ABOUT YOUR...?

Mood	①②③④⑤⑥⑦⑧⑨⑩
Energy Levels	①②③④⑤⑥⑦⑧⑨⑩
Mental Clarity	①②③④⑤⑥⑦⑧⑨⑩

PAIN & SYMPTOM DETAILS

	am	pm	front	back	other
_____	☐	☐			☐ Nausea
_____	☐	☐			☐ Diarrhea
_____	☐	☐			☐ Vomiting
_____	☐	☐			☐ Sore throat
_____	☐	☐			☐ Congestion
_____	☐	☐			☐ Coughing
_____	☐	☐			☐ Chills
_____	☐	☐			☐ Fever

SLEEP

hours   *quality*
_____   ① ② ③ ④ ⑤

STRESS LEVELS

None	Low	Medium	High	Max	@$#%!

WEATHER

☐ Cold   ☐ Mild   ☐ Hot
☐ Dry   ☐ Humid   ☐ Wet
Allergen Levels: _____
BM Pressure: _____

EXERCISE

☐ Heck yes, I worked out.
☐ I managed to exercise a bit.
☐ No, I haven't exercised at all.
☐ I did some stuff, and that counts.

DETAILS

FOOD / MEDICATION

Food / Drinks

Meds / Supplements	Time	Dose

☐ usual daily medication

Notes

I am grateful for...

HOW ARE YOU *Feeling today?*

😍 Amazing!	🙂 Meh
😁 Great	😠 Not good
🙂 Good	😵 Terrible!

RATE YOUR PAIN LEVEL

① ② ③ ④ ⑤ ⑥ ⑦ ⑧ ⑨ ⑩

WHAT ABOUT YOUR...?

Mood	① ② ③ ④ ⑤ ⑥ ⑦ ⑧ ⑨ ⑩
Energy Levels	① ② ③ ④ ⑤ ⑥ ⑦ ⑧ ⑨ ⑩
Mental Clarity	① ② ③ ④ ⑤ ⑥ ⑦ ⑧ ⑨ ⑩

PAIN & SYMPTOM DETAILS

	am	pm	front	back	other
_____	☐	☐			☐ Nausea
_____	☐	☐			☐ Diarrhea
_____	☐	☐			☐ Vomiting
_____	☐	☐			☐ Sore throat
_____	☐	☐			☐ Congestion
_____	☐	☐			☐ Coughing
_____	☐	☐			☐ Chills
_____	☐	☐			☐ Fever

SLEEP

hours
_____

quality
① ② ③ ④ ⑤

STRESS LEVELS

None	Low	Medium	High	Max	@$#%!

WEATHER

☐ Cold   ☐ Mild   ☐ Hot
☐ Dry   ☐ Humid   ☐ Wet

Allergen Levels: _____
BM Pressure: _____

EXERCISE

☐ Heck yes, I worked out.
☐ I managed to exercise a bit.
☐ No, I haven't exercised at all.
☐ I did some stuff, and that counts.

DETAILS

FOOD / MEDICATION

Food / Drinks	Meds / Supplements	Time	Dose

☐ usual daily medication

Notes
_____

I am grateful for...

M T W T F S S | DATE:

HOW ARE YOU *Feeling today?*

😍 Amazing!	🙂 Meh
😁 Great	😠 Not good
🙂 Good	😖 Terrible!

RATE YOUR PAIN LEVEL

① ② ③ ④ ⑤ ⑥ ⑦ ⑧ ⑨ ⑩

WHAT ABOUT YOUR...?

Mood	①	②	③	④	⑤	⑥	⑦	⑧	⑨	⑩
Energy Levels	①	②	③	④	⑤	⑥	⑦	⑧	⑨	⑩
Mental Clarity	①	②	③	④	⑤	⑥	⑦	⑧	⑨	⑩

PAIN & SYMPTOM DETAILS

	am	pm	front	back	other
	☐	☐			☐ Nausea
	☐	☐			☐ Diarrhea
	☐	☐			☐ Vomiting
	☐	☐			☐ Sore throat
	☐	☐			☐ Congestion
	☐	☐			☐ Coughing
	☐	☐			☐ Chills
	☐	☐			☐ Fever

SLEEP

hours _____   quality ① ② ③ ④ ⑤

STRESS LEVELS

None	Low	Medium	High	Max	@$#%!

WEATHER

☐ Cold   ☐ Mild   ☐ Hot
☐ Dry   ☐ Humid   ☐ Wet
Allergen Levels: _____
BM Pressure: _____

EXERCISE

☐ Heck yes, I worked out.
☐ I managed to exercise a bit.
☐ No, I haven't exercised at all.
☐ I did some stuff, and that counts.

DETAILS

FOOD / MEDICATION

Food / Drinks

Meds / Supplements	Time	Dose

☐ usual daily medication

Notes

I am grateful for...

M T W T F S S

DATE:

HOW ARE YOU Feeling today?

Amazing!	Meh
Great	Not good
Good	Terrible!

RATE YOUR PAIN LEVEL

① ② ③ ④ ⑤ ⑥ ⑦ ⑧ ⑨ ⑩

WHAT ABOUT YOUR...?

Mood	① ② ③ ④ ⑤ ⑥ ⑦ ⑧ ⑨ ⑩
Energy Levels	① ② ③ ④ ⑤ ⑥ ⑦ ⑧ ⑨ ⑩
Mental Clarity	① ② ③ ④ ⑤ ⑥ ⑦ ⑧ ⑨ ⑩

PAIN & SYMPTOM DETAILS

	am	pm	front	back	other
	☐	☐			☐ Nausea
	☐	☐			☐ Diarrhea
	☐	☐			☐ Vomiting
	☐	☐			☐ Sore throat
	☐	☐			☐ Congestion
	☐	☐			☐ Coughing
	☐	☐			☐ Chills
	☐	☐			☐ Fever

SLEEP

hours
_____

quality
① ② ③ ④ ⑤

STRESS LEVELS

None	Low	Medium	High	Max	@$#%!

WEATHER

☐ Cold ☐ Mild ☐ Hot
☐ Dry ☐ Humid ☐ Wet

Allergen Levels: _____
BM Pressure: _____

EXERCISE

☐ Heck yes, I worked out.
☐ I managed to exercise a bit.
☐ No, I haven't exercised at all.
☐ I did some stuff, and that counts.

DETAILS

FOOD / MEDICATION

Food / Drinks

Meds / Supplements	Time	Dose

☐ usual daily medication

Notes
_____
_____

I am grateful for...

HOW ARE YOU *Feeling today?*

😍 Amazing!	🙂 Meh
😁 Great	😠 Not good
🙂 Good	😣 Terrible!

RATE YOUR PAIN LEVEL

① ② ③ ④ ⑤ ⑥ ⑦ ⑧ ⑨ ⑩

WHAT ABOUT YOUR...?

Mood	① ② ③ ④ ⑤ ⑥ ⑦ ⑧ ⑨ ⑩
Energy Levels	① ② ③ ④ ⑤ ⑥ ⑦ ⑧ ⑨ ⑩
Mental Clarity	① ② ③ ④ ⑤ ⑥ ⑦ ⑧ ⑨ ⑩

PAIN & SYMPTOM DETAILS

	am	pm	front	back	other
_____	☐	☐			☐ Nausea
_____	☐	☐			☐ Diarrhea
_____	☐	☐			☐ Vomiting
_____	☐	☐			☐ Sore throat
_____	☐	☐			☐ Congestion
_____	☐	☐			☐ Coughing
_____	☐	☐			☐ Chills
_____	☐	☐			☐ Fever

SLEEP

hours _____   *quality* ① ② ③ ④ ⑤

STRESS LEVELS

None	Low	Medium	High	Max	@$#%!

WEATHER

☐ Cold   ☐ Mild   ☐ Hot
☐ Dry   ☐ Humid   ☐ Wet
Allergen Levels: _____
BM Pressure: _____

EXERCISE

☐ Heck yes, I worked out.
☐ I managed to exercise a bit.
☐ No, I haven't exercised at all.
☐ I did some stuff, and that counts.

DETAILS

FOOD / MEDICATION

Food / Drinks

Meds / Supplements	Time	Dose

☐ usual daily medication

Notes
_____
_____

I am grateful for...
_____

M T W T F S S   DATE:

HOW ARE YOU *Feeling today?*

😍 Amazing!	🙂 Meh
😁 Great	😖 Not good
😊 Good	😫 Terrible!

RATE YOUR PAIN LEVEL

① ② ③ ④ ⑤ ⑥ ⑦ ⑧ ⑨ ⑩

WHAT ABOUT YOUR...?

Mood	① ② ③ ④ ⑤ ⑥ ⑦ ⑧ ⑨ ⑩
Energy Levels	① ② ③ ④ ⑤ ⑥ ⑦ ⑧ ⑨ ⑩
Mental Clarity	① ② ③ ④ ⑤ ⑥ ⑦ ⑧ ⑨ ⑩

PAIN & SYMPTOM DETAILS

	am	pm	*front*	*back*	*other*
_____	☐	☐			☐ Nausea
_____	☐	☐			☐ Diarrhea
_____	☐	☐			☐ Vomiting
_____	☐	☐			☐ Sore throat
_____	☐	☐			☐ Congestion
_____	☐	☐			☐ Coughing
_____	☐	☐			☐ Chills
_____	☐	☐			☐ Fever

SLEEP

hours
_____

quality
① ② ③ ④ ⑤

STRESS LEVELS

None	Low	Medium	High	Max	@$#%!

WEATHER

☐ Cold   ☐ Mild   ☐ Hot
☐ Dry   ☐ Humid ☐ Wet

Allergen Levels: _____
BM Pressure: _____

EXERCISE

☐ Heck yes, I worked out.
☐ I managed to exercise a bit.
☐ No, I haven't exercised at all.
☐ I did some stuff, and that counts.

DETAILS

FOOD / MEDICATION

Food / Drinks

Meds / Supplements	Time	Dose

☐ usual daily medication

Notes
_____
_____

I am grateful for...
_____

HOW ARE YOU Feeling today?

Amazing!	Meh
Great	Not good
Good	Terrible!

RATE YOUR PAIN LEVEL

① ② ③ ④ ⑤ ⑥ ⑦ ⑧ ⑨ ⑩

WHAT ABOUT YOUR...?

Mood	① ② ③ ④ ⑤ ⑥ ⑦ ⑧ ⑨ ⑩
Energy Levels	① ② ③ ④ ⑤ ⑥ ⑦ ⑧ ⑨ ⑩
Mental Clarity	① ② ③ ④ ⑤ ⑥ ⑦ ⑧ ⑨ ⑩

PAIN & SYMPTOM DETAILS

	am	pm	front	back	other
	☐	☐			☐ Nausea
	☐	☐			☐ Diarrhea
	☐	☐			☐ Vomiting
	☐	☐			☐ Sore throat
	☐	☐			☐ Congestion
	☐	☐			☐ Coughing
	☐	☐			☐ Chills
	☐	☐			☐ Fever

SLEEP

hours _____   quality ① ② ③ ④ ⑤

STRESS LEVELS

| None | Low | Medium | High | Max | @$#%! |

WEATHER

☐ Cold   ☐ Mild   ☐ Hot
☐ Dry   ☐ Humid   ☐ Wet
Allergen Levels: _____
BM Pressure: _____

EXERCISE

☐ Heck yes, I worked out.
☐ I managed to exercise a bit.
☐ No, I haven't exercised at all.
☐ I did some stuff, and that counts.

DETAILS

FOOD / MEDICATION

Food / Drinks

Meds / Supplements	Time	Dose

☐ usual daily medication

Notes

I am grateful for...

HOW ARE YOU *Feeling today?*

😍 Amazing!	🙂 Meh
😁 Great	😠 Not good
🙂 Good	😖 Terrible!

RATE YOUR PAIN LEVEL

① ② ③ ④ ⑤ ⑥ ⑦ ⑧ ⑨ ⑩

WHAT ABOUT YOUR...?

Mood	① ② ③ ④ ⑤ ⑥ ⑦ ⑧ ⑨ ⑩
Energy Levels	① ② ③ ④ ⑤ ⑥ ⑦ ⑧ ⑨ ⑩
Mental Clarity	① ② ③ ④ ⑤ ⑥ ⑦ ⑧ ⑨ ⑩

PAIN & SYMPTOM DETAILS

	am	pm	front	back	other
	☐	☐			☐ Nausea
	☐	☐			☐ Diarrhea
	☐	☐			☐ Vomiting
	☐	☐			☐ Sore throat
	☐	☐			☐ Congestion
	☐	☐			☐ Coughing
	☐	☐			☐ Chills
	☐	☐			☐ Fever

SLEEP

hours _____ *quality* ① ② ③ ④ ⑤

STRESS LEVELS

None	Low	Medium	High	Max	@$#%!

WEATHER

☐ Cold ☐ Mild ☐ Hot
☐ Dry ☐ Humid ☐ Wet
Allergen Levels: _____
BM Pressure: _____

EXERCISE

☐ Heck yes, I worked out.
☐ I managed to exercise a bit.
☐ No, I haven't exercised at all.
☐ I did some stuff, and that counts.

DETAILS

FOOD / MEDICATION

Food / Drinks

Meds / Supplements	Time	Dose

☐ usual daily medication

Notes
_____
_____

I am grateful for…

HOW ARE YOU
Feeling today?

Amazing!	Meh
Great	Not good
Good	Terrible!

RATE YOUR PAIN LEVEL

① ② ③ ④ ⑤ ⑥ ⑦ ⑧ ⑨ ⑩

WHAT ABOUT YOUR...?

Mood	① ② ③ ④ ⑤ ⑥ ⑦ ⑧ ⑨ ⑩
Energy Levels	① ② ③ ④ ⑤ ⑥ ⑦ ⑧ ⑨ ⑩
Mental Clarity	① ② ③ ④ ⑤ ⑥ ⑦ ⑧ ⑨ ⑩

PAIN & SYMPTOM DETAILS

	am	pm	front	back	other
	☐	☐			☐ Nausea
	☐	☐			☐ Diarrhea
	☐	☐			☐ Vomiting
	☐	☐			☐ Sore throat
	☐	☐			☐ Congestion
	☐	☐			☐ Coughing
	☐	☐			☐ Chills
	☐	☐			☐ Fever

SLEEP

hours _____

quality ① ② ③ ④ ⑤

STRESS LEVELS

None	Low	Medium	High	Max	@$#%!

WEATHER

☐ Cold   ☐ Mild   ☐ Hot
☐ Dry   ☐ Humid ☐ Wet

Allergen Levels: _____
BM Pressure: _____

EXERCISE

☐ Heck yes, I worked out.
☐ I managed to exercise a bit.
☐ No, I haven't exercised at all.
☐ I did some stuff, and that counts.

DETAILS

FOOD / MEDICATION

Food / Drinks

Meds / Supplements	Time	Dose

☐ usual daily medication

Notes

I am grateful for...

HOW ARE YOU *Feeling today?*

Amazing!	Meh
Great	Not good
Good	Terrible!

RATE YOUR PAIN LEVEL

① ② ③ ④ ⑤ ⑥ ⑦ ⑧ ⑨ ⑩

WHAT ABOUT YOUR...?

Mood	① ② ③ ④ ⑤ ⑥ ⑦ ⑧ ⑨ ⑩
Energy Levels	① ② ③ ④ ⑤ ⑥ ⑦ ⑧ ⑨ ⑩
Mental Clarity	① ② ③ ④ ⑤ ⑥ ⑦ ⑧ ⑨ ⑩

PAIN & SYMPTOM DETAILS

	am	pm	*front*	*back*	*other*
	☐	☐			☐ Nausea
	☐	☐			☐ Diarrhea
	☐	☐			☐ Vomiting
	☐	☐			☐ Sore throat
	☐	☐			☐ Congestion
	☐	☐			☐ Coughing
	☐	☐			☐ Chills
	☐	☐			☐ Fever

SLEEP

hours _____

quality ① ② ③ ④ ⑤

STRESS LEVELS

None	Low	Medium	High	Max	@$#%!

WEATHER

☐ Cold ☐ Mild ☐ Hot
☐ Dry ☐ Humid ☐ Wet
Allergen Levels: _____
BM Pressure: _____

EXERCISE

☐ Heck yes, I worked out.
☐ I managed to exercise a bit.
☐ No, I haven't exercised at all.
☐ I did some stuff, and that counts.

DETAILS

FOOD / MEDICATION

Food / Drinks

Meds / Supplements	Time	Dose

☐ usual daily medication

Notes
_____
_____

I am grateful for...

HOW ARE YOU *Feeling today?*

😍 Amazing!	🙂 Meh
😁 Great	😠 Not good
🙂 Good	😫 Terrible!

RATE YOUR PAIN LEVEL

① ② ③ ④ ⑤ ⑥ ⑦ ⑧ ⑨ ⑩

WHAT ABOUT YOUR...?

Mood	① ② ③ ④ ⑤ ⑥ ⑦ ⑧ ⑨ ⑩
Energy Levels	① ② ③ ④ ⑤ ⑥ ⑦ ⑧ ⑨ ⑩
Mental Clarity	① ② ③ ④ ⑤ ⑥ ⑦ ⑧ ⑨ ⑩

PAIN & SYMPTOM DETAILS

	am	pm	front	back	other
_____	☐	☐			☐ Nausea
_____	☐	☐			☐ Diarrhea
_____	☐	☐			☐ Vomiting
_____	☐	☐			☐ Sore throat
_____	☐	☐			☐ Congestion
_____	☐	☐			☐ Coughing
_____	☐	☐			☐ Chills
_____	☐	☐			☐ Fever

SLEEP

hours
_____

quality
① ② ③ ④ ⑤

STRESS LEVELS

None	Low	Medium	High	Max	@$#%!

WEATHER

☐ Cold   ☐ Mild   ☐ Hot
☐ Dry   ☐ Humid   ☐ Wet

Allergen Levels: _____
BM Pressure: _____

EXERCISE

☐ Heck yes, I worked out.
☐ I managed to exercise a bit.
☐ No, I haven't exercised at all.
☐ I did some stuff, and that counts.

DETAILS

FOOD / MEDICATION

Food / Drinks

Meds / Supplements	Time	Dose

☐ usual daily medication

Notes
_____

I am grateful for...
_____

M T W T F S S   DATE:

HOW ARE YOU *Feeling today?*

Amazing!	Meh
Great	Not good
Good	Terrible!

RATE YOUR PAIN LEVEL

① ② ③ ④ ⑤ ⑥ ⑦ ⑧ ⑨ ⑩

WHAT ABOUT YOUR...?

Mood	① ② ③ ④ ⑤ ⑥ ⑦ ⑧ ⑨ ⑩
Energy Levels	① ② ③ ④ ⑤ ⑥ ⑦ ⑧ ⑨ ⑩
Mental Clarity	① ② ③ ④ ⑤ ⑥ ⑦ ⑧ ⑨ ⑩

PAIN & SYMPTOM DETAILS

	am	pm	*front*	*back*	*other*
_____	☐	☐			☐ Nausea
_____	☐	☐			☐ Diarrhea
_____	☐	☐			☐ Vomiting
_____	☐	☐			☐ Sore throat
_____	☐	☐			☐ Congestion
_____	☐	☐			☐ Coughing
_____	☐	☐			☐ Chills
_____	☐	☐			☐ Fever

SLEEP

hours _____   *quality* ① ② ③ ④ ⑤

STRESS LEVELS

None	Low	Medium	High	Max	@$#%!

WEATHER

☐ Cold   ☐ Mild   ☐ Hot
☐ Dry   ☐ Humid   ☐ Wet
Allergen Levels: _____
BM Pressure: _____

EXERCISE

☐ Heck yes, I worked out.
☐ I managed to exercise a bit.
☐ No, I haven't exercised at all.
☐ I did some stuff, and that counts.

DETAILS

FOOD / MEDICATION

Food / Drinks

Meds / Supplements	Time	Dose

☐ usual daily medication

Notes
_____
_____

I am grateful for...

HOW ARE YOU *Feeling today?*

Amazing!	Meh
Great	Not good
Good	Terrible!

RATE YOUR PAIN LEVEL

① ② ③ ④ ⑤ ⑥ ⑦ ⑧ ⑨ ⑩

WHAT ABOUT YOUR...?

Mood	① ② ③ ④ ⑤ ⑥ ⑦ ⑧ ⑨ ⑩
Energy Levels	① ② ③ ④ ⑤ ⑥ ⑦ ⑧ ⑨ ⑩
Mental Clarity	① ② ③ ④ ⑤ ⑥ ⑦ ⑧ ⑨ ⑩

PAIN & SYMPTOM DETAILS

	am	pm	*front*	*back*	*other*
_____	☐	☐			☐ Nausea
_____	☐	☐			☐ Diarrhea
_____	☐	☐			☐ Vomiting
_____	☐	☐			☐ Sore throat
_____	☐	☐			☐ Congestion
_____	☐	☐			☐ Coughing
_____	☐	☐			☐ Chills
_____	☐	☐			☐ Fever

SLEEP

hours _____   *quality* ① ② ③ ④ ⑤

STRESS LEVELS

None	Low	Medium	High	Max	@$#%!

WEATHER

☐ Cold   ☐ Mild   ☐ Hot
☐ Dry   ☐ Humid ☐ Wet

Allergen Levels: _____
BM Pressure: _____

EXERCISE

☐ Heck yes, I worked out.
☐ I managed to exercise a bit.
☐ No, I haven't exercised at all.
☐ I did some stuff, and that counts.

DETAILS

FOOD / MEDICATION

Food / Drinks

Meds / Supplements	Time	Dose

☐ usual daily medication

Notes
_____
_____

I am grateful for...
_____

HOW ARE YOU *Feeling today?*

😍 Amazing!	🙂 Meh
😁 Great	😠 Not good
🙂 Good	😖 Terrible!

RATE YOUR PAIN LEVEL

① ② ③ ④ ⑤ ⑥ ⑦ ⑧ ⑨ ⑩

WHAT ABOUT YOUR...?

Mood	① ② ③ ④ ⑤ ⑥ ⑦ ⑧ ⑨ ⑩
Energy Levels	① ② ③ ④ ⑤ ⑥ ⑦ ⑧ ⑨ ⑩
Mental Clarity	① ② ③ ④ ⑤ ⑥ ⑦ ⑧ ⑨ ⑩

PAIN & SYMPTOM DETAILS

	am	pm	*front*	*back*	*other*
_____	☐	☐			☐ Nausea
_____	☐	☐			☐ Diarrhea
_____	☐	☐			☐ Vomiting
_____	☐	☐			☐ Sore throat
_____	☐	☐			☐ Congestion
_____	☐	☐			☐ Coughing
_____	☐	☐			☐ Chills
_____	☐	☐			☐ Fever

SLEEP

hours
_____

quality
① ② ③ ④ ⑤

STRESS LEVELS

None	Low	Medium	High	Max	@$#%!

WEATHER

☐ Cold　☐ Mild　☐ Hot
☐ Dry　☐ Humid　☐ Wet

Allergen Levels: _____
BM Pressure: _____

EXERCISE

☐ Heck yes, I worked out.
☐ I managed to exercise a bit.
☐ No, I haven't exercised at all.
☐ I did some stuff, and that counts.

DETAILS

FOOD / MEDICATION

Food / Drinks	Meds / Supplements	Time	Dose
	☐ usual daily medication		

Notes
_____
_____

I am grateful for…

M T W T F S S   DATE:

HOW ARE YOU Feeling today?

Amazing!	Meh
Great	Not good
Good	Terrible!

RATE YOUR PAIN LEVEL

① ② ③ ④ ⑤ ⑥ ⑦ ⑧ ⑨ ⑩

WHAT ABOUT YOUR...?

Mood	① ② ③ ④ ⑤ ⑥ ⑦ ⑧ ⑨ ⑩
Energy Levels	① ② ③ ④ ⑤ ⑥ ⑦ ⑧ ⑨ ⑩
Mental Clarity	① ② ③ ④ ⑤ ⑥ ⑦ ⑧ ⑨ ⑩

PAIN & SYMPTOM DETAILS

	am	pm	front	back	other
	☐	☐			☐ Nausea
	☐	☐			☐ Diarrhea
	☐	☐			☐ Vomiting
	☐	☐			☐ Sore throat
	☐	☐			☐ Congestion
	☐	☐			☐ Coughing
	☐	☐			☐ Chills
	☐	☐			☐ Fever

SLEEP

hours _____

quality ① ② ③ ④ ⑤

STRESS LEVELS

None	Low	Medium	High	Max	@$#%!

WEATHER

☐ Cold   ☐ Mild   ☐ Hot
☐ Dry   ☐ Humid ☐ Wet
Allergen Levels: _____
BM Pressure: _____

EXERCISE

☐ Heck yes, I worked out.
☐ I managed to exercise a bit.
☐ No, I haven't exercised at all.
☐ I did some stuff, and that counts.

DETAILS

FOOD / MEDICATION

Food / Drinks

Meds / Supplements	Time	Dose

☐ usual daily medication

Notes

I am grateful for...

M T W T F S S   DATE:

HOW ARE YOU Feeling today?

Amazing!	Meh
Great	Not good
Good	Terrible!

RATE YOUR PAIN LEVEL

① ② ③ ④ ⑤ ⑥ ⑦ ⑧ ⑨ ⑩

WHAT ABOUT YOUR...?

Mood	① ② ③ ④ ⑤ ⑥ ⑦ ⑧ ⑨ ⑩
Energy Levels	① ② ③ ④ ⑤ ⑥ ⑦ ⑧ ⑨ ⑩
Mental Clarity	① ② ③ ④ ⑤ ⑥ ⑦ ⑧ ⑨ ⑩

PAIN & SYMPTOM DETAILS

	am	pm	front	back	other
	☐	☐			☐ Nausea
	☐	☐			☐ Diarrhea
	☐	☐			☐ Vomiting
	☐	☐			☐ Sore throat
	☐	☐			☐ Congestion
	☐	☐			☐ Coughing
	☐	☐			☐ Chills
	☐	☐			☐ Fever

SLEEP

hours   quality
_____   ① ② ③ ④ ⑤

STRESS LEVELS

None	Low	Medium	High	Max	@$#%!

WEATHER

☐ Cold   ☐ Mild   ☐ Hot
☐ Dry   ☐ Humid   ☐ Wet
Allergen Levels: _____
BM Pressure: _____

EXERCISE

☐ Heck yes, I worked out.
☐ I managed to exercise a bit.
☐ No, I haven't exercised at all.
☐ I did some stuff, and that counts.

DETAILS

FOOD / MEDICATION

Food / Drinks	Meds / Supplements	Time	Dose

☐ usual daily medication

Notes
_____
_____

I am grateful for...

M T W T F S S   DATE:

HOW ARE YOU *Feeling today?*

Amazing!	Meh
Great	Not good
Good	Terrible!

RATE YOUR PAIN LEVEL

① ② ③ ④ ⑤ ⑥ ⑦ ⑧ ⑨ ⑩

WHAT ABOUT YOUR...?

Mood	① ② ③ ④ ⑤ ⑥ ⑦ ⑧ ⑨ ⑩
Energy Levels	① ② ③ ④ ⑤ ⑥ ⑦ ⑧ ⑨ ⑩
Mental Clarity	① ② ③ ④ ⑤ ⑥ ⑦ ⑧ ⑨ ⑩

PAIN & SYMPTOM DETAILS

	am	pm	front	back	other
	☐	☐			☐ Nausea
	☐	☐			☐ Diarrhea
	☐	☐			☐ Vomiting
	☐	☐			☐ Sore throat
	☐	☐			☐ Congestion
	☐	☐			☐ Coughing
	☐	☐			☐ Chills
	☐	☐			☐ Fever

SLEEP

hours _____   *quality* ① ② ③ ④ ⑤

STRESS LEVELS

None	Low	Medium	High	Max	@$#%!

WEATHER

☐ Cold   ☐ Mild   ☐ Hot
☐ Dry   ☐ Humid   ☐ Wet
Allergen Levels: _____
BM Pressure: _____

EXERCISE

☐ Heck yes, I worked out.
☐ I managed to exercise a bit.
☐ No, I haven't exercised at all.
☐ I did some stuff, and that counts.

DETAILS

FOOD / MEDICATION

Food / Drinks

Meds / Supplements	Time	Dose

☐ usual daily medication

Notes

I am grateful for…

M T W T F S S

DATE:

HOW ARE YOU *Feeling today?*

😍 Amazing!	🙂 Meh
😁 Great	😖 Not good
😊 Good	😵 Terrible!

RATE YOUR PAIN LEVEL

① ② ③ ④ ⑤ ⑥ ⑦ ⑧ ⑨ ⑩

WHAT ABOUT YOUR...?

Mood	① ② ③ ④ ⑤ ⑥ ⑦ ⑧ ⑨ ⑩
Energy Levels	① ② ③ ④ ⑤ ⑥ ⑦ ⑧ ⑨ ⑩
Mental Clarity	① ② ③ ④ ⑤ ⑥ ⑦ ⑧ ⑨ ⑩

PAIN & SYMPTOM DETAILS

	am	pm	*front*	*back*	*other*
_____	☐	☐			☐ Nausea
_____	☐	☐			☐ Diarrhea
_____	☐	☐			☐ Vomiting
_____	☐	☐			☐ Sore throat
_____	☐	☐			☐ Congestion
_____	☐	☐			☐ Coughing
_____	☐	☐			☐ Chills
_____	☐	☐			☐ Fever

SLEEP

hours
_____

quality
① ② ③ ④ ⑤

STRESS LEVELS

None	Low	Medium	High	Max	@$#%!

WEATHER

☐ Cold ☐ Mild ☐ Hot
☐ Dry ☐ Humid ☐ Wet

Allergen Levels: _____
BM Pressure: _____

EXERCISE

☐ Heck yes, I worked out.
☐ I managed to exercise a bit.
☐ No, I haven't exercised at all.
☐ I did some stuff, and that counts.

DETAILS

FOOD / MEDICATION

Food / Drinks

Meds / Supplements	Time	Dose

☐ usual daily medication

Notes
_____
_____

I am grateful for...

M T W T F S S

DATE:

HOW ARE YOU Feeling today?

Amazing!	Meh
Great	Not good
Good	Terrible!

RATE YOUR PAIN LEVEL

① ② ③ ④ ⑤ ⑥ ⑦ ⑧ ⑨ ⑩

WHAT ABOUT YOUR...?

Mood	① ② ③ ④ ⑤ ⑥ ⑦ ⑧ ⑨ ⑩
Energy Levels	① ② ③ ④ ⑤ ⑥ ⑦ ⑧ ⑨ ⑩
Mental Clarity	① ② ③ ④ ⑤ ⑥ ⑦ ⑧ ⑨ ⑩

PAIN & SYMPTOM DETAILS

| | am | pm | front | back | other |

other
- ☐ Nausea
- ☐ Diarrhea
- ☐ Vomiting
- ☐ Sore throat
- ☐ Congestion
- ☐ Coughing
- ☐ Chills
- ☐ Fever

SLEEP

hours _____

quality ① ② ③ ④ ⑤

STRESS LEVELS

| None | Low | Medium | High | Max | @$#%! |

WEATHER

- ☐ Cold   ☐ Mild   ☐ Hot
- ☐ Dry   ☐ Humid   ☐ Wet

Allergen Levels: _____

BM Pressure: _____

EXERCISE

- ☐ Heck yes, I worked out.
- ☐ I managed to exercise a bit.
- ☐ No, I haven't exercised at all.
- ☐ I did some stuff, and that counts.

DETAILS

FOOD / MEDICATION

Food / Drinks

Meds / Supplements	Time	Dose

☐ usual daily medication

Notes

I am grateful for…

HOW ARE YOU *Feeling today?*

😍 Amazing!	🙂 Meh
😁 Great	😣 Not good
😊 Good	😖 Terrible!

RATE YOUR PAIN LEVEL

① ② ③ ④ ⑤ ⑥ ⑦ ⑧ ⑨ ⑩

WHAT ABOUT YOUR...?

Mood	① ② ③ ④ ⑤ ⑥ ⑦ ⑧ ⑨ ⑩
Energy Levels	① ② ③ ④ ⑤ ⑥ ⑦ ⑧ ⑨ ⑩
Mental Clarity	① ② ③ ④ ⑤ ⑥ ⑦ ⑧ ⑨ ⑩

PAIN & SYMPTOM DETAILS

	am	pm	*front*	*back*	*other*
_____	☐	☐			☐ Nausea
_____	☐	☐			☐ Diarrhea
_____	☐	☐			☐ Vomiting
_____	☐	☐			☐ Sore throat
_____	☐	☐			☐ Congestion
_____	☐	☐			☐ Coughing
_____	☐	☐			☐ Chills
_____	☐	☐			☐ Fever

SLEEP

hours
_____

quality
① ② ③ ④ ⑤

STRESS LEVELS

None	Low	Medium	High	Max	@$#%!

WEATHER

☐ Cold ☐ Mild ☐ Hot
☐ Dry ☐ Humid ☐ Wet
Allergen Levels: _____
BM Pressure: _____

EXERCISE

☐ Heck yes, I worked out.
☐ I managed to exercise a bit.
☐ No, I haven't exercised at all.
☐ I did some stuff, and that counts.

DETAILS

FOOD / MEDICATION

Food / Drinks

Meds / Supplements	Time	Dose

☐ usual daily medication

Notes
_____

I am grateful for...
_____

HOW ARE YOU *Feeling today?*

Amazing!	Meh
Great	Not good
Good	Terrible!

RATE YOUR PAIN LEVEL

① ② ③ ④ ⑤ ⑥ ⑦ ⑧ ⑨ ⑩

WHAT ABOUT YOUR...?

Mood	① ② ③ ④ ⑤ ⑥ ⑦ ⑧ ⑨ ⑩
Energy Levels	① ② ③ ④ ⑤ ⑥ ⑦ ⑧ ⑨ ⑩
Mental Clarity	① ② ③ ④ ⑤ ⑥ ⑦ ⑧ ⑨ ⑩

PAIN & SYMPTOM DETAILS

	am	pm	front	back	other
_____	☐	☐			☐ Nausea
_____	☐	☐			☐ Diarrhea
_____	☐	☐			☐ Vomiting
_____	☐	☐			☐ Sore throat
_____	☐	☐			☐ Congestion
_____	☐	☐			☐ Coughing
_____	☐	☐			☐ Chills
_____	☐	☐			☐ Fever

SLEEP

hours   *quality*
_____   ① ② ③ ④ ⑤

STRESS LEVELS

| None | Low | Medium | High | Max | @$#%! |

WEATHER

☐ Cold   ☐ Mild   ☐ Hot
☐ Dry   ☐ Humid   ☐ Wet
Allergen Levels: _____
BM Pressure: _____

EXERCISE

☐ Heck yes, I worked out.
☐ I managed to exercise a bit.
☐ No, I haven't exercised at all.
☐ I did some stuff, and that counts.

DETAILS

FOOD / MEDICATION

Food / Drinks

Meds / Supplements	Time	Dose

☐ usual daily medication

Notes
_____

I am grateful for...

M T W T F S S   DATE:

HOW ARE YOU *Feeling today?*

Amazing!	Meh
Great	Not good
Good	Terrible!

RATE YOUR PAIN LEVEL

① ② ③ ④ ⑤ ⑥ ⑦ ⑧ ⑨ ⑩

WHAT ABOUT YOUR...?

Mood	① ② ③ ④ ⑤ ⑥ ⑦ ⑧ ⑨ ⑩
Energy Levels	① ② ③ ④ ⑤ ⑥ ⑦ ⑧ ⑨ ⑩
Mental Clarity	① ② ③ ④ ⑤ ⑥ ⑦ ⑧ ⑨ ⑩

PAIN & SYMPTOM DETAILS

am	pm	*front*	*back*	*other*
☐	☐			☐ Nausea
☐	☐			☐ Diarrhea
☐	☐			☐ Vomiting
☐	☐			☐ Sore throat
☐	☐			☐ Congestion
☐	☐			☐ Coughing
☐	☐			☐ Chills
☐	☐			☐ Fever

SLEEP

hours _____   *quality* ① ② ③ ④ ⑤

STRESS LEVELS

None	Low	Medium	High	Max	@$#%!

WEATHER

☐ Cold   ☐ Mild   ☐ Hot
☐ Dry   ☐ Humid ☐ Wet

Allergen Levels: _____
BM Pressure: _____

EXERCISE

☐ Heck yes, I worked out.
☐ I managed to exercise a bit.
☐ No, I haven't exercised at all.
☐ I did some stuff, and that counts.

DETAILS

FOOD / MEDICATION

Food / Drinks

Meds / Supplements	Time	Dose

☐ usual daily medication

Notes _____

_____

I am grateful for... _____

M T W T F S S   DATE:

HOW ARE YOU *Feeling today?*

😍 Amazing!	🙂 Meh
😁 Great	😠 Not good
😊 Good	😖 Terrible!

RATE YOUR PAIN LEVEL

① ② ③ ④ ⑤ ⑥ ⑦ ⑧ ⑨ ⑩

WHAT ABOUT YOUR...?

Mood	① ② ③ ④ ⑤ ⑥ ⑦ ⑧ ⑨ ⑩
Energy Levels	① ② ③ ④ ⑤ ⑥ ⑦ ⑧ ⑨ ⑩
Mental Clarity	① ② ③ ④ ⑤ ⑥ ⑦ ⑧ ⑨ ⑩

PAIN & SYMPTOM DETAILS

	am	pm				other
	☐	☐	*front*	*back*		☐ Nausea
	☐	☐				☐ Diarrhea
	☐	☐				☐ Vomiting
	☐	☐				☐ Sore throat
	☐	☐				☐ Congestion
	☐	☐				☐ Coughing
	☐	☐				☐ Chills
	☐	☐				☐ Fever

SLEEP

hours _____   *quality* ① ② ③ ④ ⑤

STRESS LEVELS

None	Low	Medium	High	Max	@$#%!

WEATHER

☐ Cold   ☐ Mild   ☐ Hot
☐ Dry   ☐ Humid   ☐ Wet
Allergen Levels: _____
BM Pressure: _____

EXERCISE

☐ Heck yes, I worked out.
☐ I managed to exercise a bit.
☐ No, I haven't exercised at all.
☐ I did some stuff, and that counts.

DETAILS

FOOD / MEDICATION

Food / Drinks	Meds / Supplements	Time	Dose

☐ usual daily medication

Notes

I am grateful for...

M T W T F S S   DATE:

HOW ARE YOU Feeling today?

Amazing!	Meh
Great	Not good
Good	Terrible!

RATE YOUR PAIN LEVEL

① ② ③ ④ ⑤ ⑥ ⑦ ⑧ ⑨ ⑩

WHAT ABOUT YOUR...?

Mood	① ② ③ ④ ⑤ ⑥ ⑦ ⑧ ⑨ ⑩
Energy Levels	① ② ③ ④ ⑤ ⑥ ⑦ ⑧ ⑨ ⑩
Mental Clarity	① ② ③ ④ ⑤ ⑥ ⑦ ⑧ ⑨ ⑩

PAIN & SYMPTOM DETAILS

	am	pm	front	back	other
_____	☐	☐			☐ Nausea
_____	☐	☐			☐ Diarrhea
_____	☐	☐			☐ Vomiting
_____	☐	☐			☐ Sore throat
_____	☐	☐			☐ Congestion
_____	☐	☐			☐ Coughing
_____	☐	☐			☐ Chills
_____	☐	☐			☐ Fever

SLEEP

hours _____

quality ① ② ③ ④ ⑤

STRESS LEVELS

None	Low	Medium	High	Max	@$#%!

WEATHER

☐ Cold ☐ Mild ☐ Hot
☐ Dry ☐ Humid ☐ Wet

Allergen Levels: _____
BM Pressure: _____

EXERCISE

☐ Heck yes, I worked out.
☐ I managed to exercise a bit.
☐ No, I haven't exercised at all.
☐ I did some stuff, and that counts.

DETAILS

FOOD / MEDICATION

Food / Drinks

Meds / Supplements	Time	Dose

☐ usual daily medication

Notes
_____
_____

I am grateful for...

M T W T F S S

DATE:

HOW ARE YOU Feeling today?

😍 Amazing!	🙂 Meh
😁 Great	😠 Not good
🙂 Good	😖 Terrible!

RATE YOUR PAIN LEVEL

① ② ③ ④ ⑤ ⑥ ⑦ ⑧ ⑨ ⑩

WHAT ABOUT YOUR...?

Mood	① ② ③ ④ ⑤ ⑥ ⑦ ⑧ ⑨ ⑩
Energy Levels	① ② ③ ④ ⑤ ⑥ ⑦ ⑧ ⑨ ⑩
Mental Clarity	① ② ③ ④ ⑤ ⑥ ⑦ ⑧ ⑨ ⑩

PAIN & SYMPTOM DETAILS

	am	pm	front	back	other
_____	☐	☐			☐ Nausea
_____	☐	☐			☐ Diarrhea
_____	☐	☐			☐ Vomiting
_____	☐	☐			☐ Sore throat
_____	☐	☐			☐ Congestion
_____	☐	☐			☐ Coughing
_____	☐	☐			☐ Chills
_____	☐	☐			☐ Fever

SLEEP

hours _____ *quality* ① ② ③ ④ ⑤

STRESS LEVELS

None	Low	Medium	High	Max	@$#%!

WEATHER

☐ Cold ☐ Mild ☐ Hot
☐ Dry ☐ Humid ☐ Wet
Allergen Levels: _____
BM Pressure: _____

EXERCISE

☐ Heck yes, I worked out.
☐ I managed to exercise a bit.
☐ No, I haven't exercised at all.
☐ I did some stuff, and that counts.

DETAILS

FOOD / MEDICATION

Food / Drinks

Meds / Supplements	Time	Dose

☐ usual daily medication

Notes
_____

I am grateful for...
_____

HOW ARE YOU *Feeling today?*

Amazing!	Meh
Great	Not good
Good	Terrible!

RATE YOUR PAIN LEVEL

① ② ③ ④ ⑤ ⑥ ⑦ ⑧ ⑨ ⑩

WHAT ABOUT YOUR...?

Mood	① ② ③ ④ ⑤ ⑥ ⑦ ⑧ ⑨ ⑩
Energy Levels	① ② ③ ④ ⑤ ⑥ ⑦ ⑧ ⑨ ⑩
Mental Clarity	① ② ③ ④ ⑤ ⑥ ⑦ ⑧ ⑨ ⑩

PAIN & SYMPTOM DETAILS

	am	pm	front	back	other
_____	☐	☐			☐ Nausea
_____	☐	☐			☐ Diarrhea
_____	☐	☐			☐ Vomiting
_____	☐	☐			☐ Sore throat
_____	☐	☐			☐ Congestion
_____	☐	☐			☐ Coughing
_____	☐	☐			☐ Chills
_____	☐	☐			☐ Fever

SLEEP

hours _____

quality ① ② ③ ④ ⑤

STRESS LEVELS

None	Low	Medium	High	Max	@$#%!

WEATHER

☐ Cold   ☐ Mild   ☐ Hot
☐ Dry   ☐ Humid ☐ Wet
Allergen Levels: _____
BM Pressure: _____

EXERCISE

☐ Heck yes, I worked out.
☐ I managed to exercise a bit.
☐ No, I haven't exercised at all.
☐ I did some stuff, and that counts.

DETAILS

FOOD / MEDICATION

Food / Drinks

Meds / Supplements	Time	Dose

☐ usual daily medication

Notes
_____
_____

I am grateful for...

HOW ARE YOU *Feeling today?*

😍 Amazing!	🙂 Meh
😁 Great	😠 Not good
😊 Good	😫 Terrible!

RATE YOUR PAIN LEVEL

① ② ③ ④ ⑤ ⑥ ⑦ ⑧ ⑨ ⑩

WHAT ABOUT YOUR...?

Mood	① ② ③ ④ ⑤ ⑥ ⑦ ⑧ ⑨ ⑩
Energy Levels	① ② ③ ④ ⑤ ⑥ ⑦ ⑧ ⑨ ⑩
Mental Clarity	① ② ③ ④ ⑤ ⑥ ⑦ ⑧ ⑨ ⑩

PAIN & SYMPTOM DETAILS

	am	pm
_____	☐	☐
_____	☐	☐
_____	☐	☐
_____	☐	☐
_____	☐	☐
_____	☐	☐
_____	☐	☐

front   *back*

other

☐ Nausea
☐ Diarrhea
☐ Vomiting
☐ Sore throat
☐ Congestion
☐ Coughing
☐ Chills
☐ Fever

SLEEP

hours   *quality*
_____   ① ② ③ ④ ⑤

STRESS LEVELS

None	Low	Medium	High	Max	@$#%!

WEATHER

☐ Cold   ☐ Mild   ☐ Hot
☐ Dry   ☐ Humid   ☐ Wet

Allergen Levels: _____
BM Pressure: _____

EXERCISE

☐ Heck yes, I worked out.
☐ I managed to exercise a bit.
☐ No, I haven't exercised at all.
☐ I did some stuff, and that counts.

DETAILS

FOOD / MEDICATION

Food / Drinks

Meds / Supplements	Time	Dose

☐ usual daily medication

Notes
_____
_____

I am grateful for...

M T W T F S S   DATE:

HOW ARE YOU *Feeling today?*

Amazing!	Meh
Great	Not good
Good	Terrible!

RATE YOUR PAIN LEVEL

① ② ③ ④ ⑤ ⑥ ⑦ ⑧ ⑨ ⑩

WHAT ABOUT YOUR...?

Mood	① ② ③ ④ ⑤ ⑥ ⑦ ⑧ ⑨ ⑩
Energy Levels	① ② ③ ④ ⑤ ⑥ ⑦ ⑧ ⑨ ⑩
Mental Clarity	① ② ③ ④ ⑤ ⑥ ⑦ ⑧ ⑨ ⑩

PAIN & SYMPTOM DETAILS

	am	pm	front	back	other
	☐	☐			☐ Nausea
	☐	☐			☐ Diarrhea
	☐	☐			☐ Vomiting
	☐	☐			☐ Sore throat
	☐	☐			☐ Congestion
	☐	☐			☐ Coughing
	☐	☐			☐ Chills
	☐	☐			☐ Fever

SLEEP

hours _____

quality ① ② ③ ④ ⑤

STRESS LEVELS

None	Low	Medium	High	Max	@$#%!

WEATHER

☐ Cold ☐ Mild ☐ Hot
☐ Dry ☐ Humid ☐ Wet

Allergen Levels: _____
BM Pressure: _____

EXERCISE

☐ Heck yes, I worked out.
☐ I managed to exercise a bit.
☐ No, I haven't exercised at all.
☐ I did some stuff, and that counts.

DETAILS

FOOD / MEDICATION

Food / Drinks

Meds / Supplements	Time	Dose

☐ usual daily medication

Notes
_____

I am grateful for...

M T W T F S S

DATE:

HOW ARE YOU Feeling today?

Amazing!	Meh
Great	Not good
Good	Terrible!

RATE YOUR PAIN LEVEL

① ② ③ ④ ⑤ ⑥ ⑦ ⑧ ⑨ ⑩

WHAT ABOUT YOUR...?

Mood	① ② ③ ④ ⑤ ⑥ ⑦ ⑧ ⑨ ⑩
Energy Levels	① ② ③ ④ ⑤ ⑥ ⑦ ⑧ ⑨ ⑩
Mental Clarity	① ② ③ ④ ⑤ ⑥ ⑦ ⑧ ⑨ ⑩

PAIN & SYMPTOM DETAILS

	am	pm	front	back	other
	☐	☐			☐ Nausea
	☐	☐			☐ Diarrhea
	☐	☐			☐ Vomiting
	☐	☐			☐ Sore throat
	☐	☐			☐ Congestion
	☐	☐			☐ Coughing
	☐	☐			☐ Chills
	☐	☐			☐ Fever

SLEEP

hours _____   *quality* ① ② ③ ④ ⑤

STRESS LEVELS

None	Low	Medium	High	Max	@$#%!

WEATHER

☐ Cold   ☐ Mild   ☐ Hot
☐ Dry   ☐ Humid   ☐ Wet
Allergen Levels: _____
BM Pressure: _____

EXERCISE

☐ Heck yes, I worked out.
☐ I managed to exercise a bit.
☐ No, I haven't exercised at all.
☐ I did some stuff, and that counts.

DETAILS

FOOD / MEDICATION

Food / Drinks

Meds / Supplements	Time	Dose

☐ usual daily medication

Notes

I am grateful for...

M T W T F S S

DATE:

HOW ARE YOU *Feeling today?*

😍 Amazing!	🙂 Meh
😁 Great	😠 Not good
😊 Good	😖 Terrible!

RATE YOUR PAIN LEVEL

① ② ③ ④ ⑤ ⑥ ⑦ ⑧ ⑨ ⑩

WHAT ABOUT YOUR...?

Mood	① ② ③ ④ ⑤ ⑥ ⑦ ⑧ ⑨ ⑩
Energy Levels	① ② ③ ④ ⑤ ⑥ ⑦ ⑧ ⑨ ⑩
Mental Clarity	① ② ③ ④ ⑤ ⑥ ⑦ ⑧ ⑨ ⑩

PAIN & SYMPTOM DETAILS

	am	pm	front	back	other
	☐	☐			☐ Nausea
	☐	☐			☐ Diarrhea
	☐	☐			☐ Vomiting
	☐	☐			☐ Sore throat
	☐	☐			☐ Congestion
	☐	☐			☐ Coughing
	☐	☐			☐ Chills
	☐	☐			☐ Fever

SLEEP

hours _____

quality ① ② ③ ④ ⑤

STRESS LEVELS

None	Low	Medium	High	Max	@$#%!

WEATHER

☐ Cold   ☐ Mild   ☐ Hot
☐ Dry   ☐ Humid   ☐ Wet

Allergen Levels: _____
BM Pressure: _____

EXERCISE

☐ Heck yes, I worked out.
☐ I managed to exercise a bit.
☐ No, I haven't exercised at all.
☐ I did some stuff, and that counts.

DETAILS

FOOD / MEDICATION

Food / Drinks

Meds / Supplements	Time	Dose

☐ usual daily medication

Notes
_____

I am grateful for...

M T W T F S S | DATE:

HOW ARE YOU *Feeling today?*

😍 Amazing!	🙂 Meh
😁 Great	😠 Not good
😊 Good	😖 Terrible!

RATE YOUR PAIN LEVEL

① ② ③ ④ ⑤ ⑥ ⑦ ⑧ ⑨ ⑩

WHAT ABOUT YOUR...?

Mood	① ② ③ ④ ⑤ ⑥ ⑦ ⑧ ⑨ ⑩
Energy Levels	① ② ③ ④ ⑤ ⑥ ⑦ ⑧ ⑨ ⑩
Mental Clarity	① ② ③ ④ ⑤ ⑥ ⑦ ⑧ ⑨ ⑩

PAIN & SYMPTOM DETAILS

	am	pm
_____	☐	☐
_____	☐	☐
_____	☐	☐
_____	☐	☐
_____	☐	☐
_____	☐	☐
_____	☐	☐
_____	☐	☐

front　　*back*

other
- ☐ Nausea
- ☐ Diarrhea
- ☐ Vomiting
- ☐ Sore throat
- ☐ Congestion
- ☐ Coughing
- ☐ Chills
- ☐ Fever

SLEEP

hours　　　　*quality*
_____　　① ② ③ ④ ⑤

STRESS LEVELS

None	Low	Medium	High	Max	@$#%!

WEATHER

- ☐ Cold　☐ Mild　☐ Hot
- ☐ Dry　☐ Humid　☐ Wet

Allergen Levels: _____
BM Pressure: _____

EXERCISE

- ☐ Heck yes, I worked out.
- ☐ I managed to exercise a bit.
- ☐ No, I haven't exercised at all.
- ☐ I did some stuff, and that counts.

DETAILS

FOOD / MEDICATION

Food / Drinks

Meds / Supplements	Time	Dose

☐ usual daily medication

Notes
_____

I am grateful for...

M T W T F S S   DATE:

HOW ARE YOU *Feeling today?*

😍 Amazing!	🙂 Meh
😁 Great	😠 Not good
😊 Good	😖 Terrible!

RATE YOUR PAIN LEVEL

① ② ③ ④ ⑤ ⑥ ⑦ ⑧ ⑨ ⑩

WHAT ABOUT YOUR...?

Mood	① ② ③ ④ ⑤ ⑥ ⑦ ⑧ ⑨ ⑩
Energy Levels	① ② ③ ④ ⑤ ⑥ ⑦ ⑧ ⑨ ⑩
Mental Clarity	① ② ③ ④ ⑤ ⑥ ⑦ ⑧ ⑨ ⑩

PAIN & SYMPTOM DETAILS

	am	pm	front	back	other
	☐	☐			☐ Nausea
	☐	☐			☐ Diarrhea
	☐	☐			☐ Vomiting
	☐	☐			☐ Sore throat
	☐	☐			☐ Congestion
	☐	☐			☐ Coughing
	☐	☐			☐ Chills
	☐	☐			☐ Fever

SLEEP

hours _____   *quality* ① ② ③ ④ ⑤

STRESS LEVELS

None	Low	Medium	High	Max	@$#%!

WEATHER

☐ Cold   ☐ Mild   ☐ Hot
☐ Dry   ☐ Humid   ☐ Wet
Allergen Levels: _____
BM Pressure: _____

EXERCISE

☐ Heck yes, I worked out.
☐ I managed to exercise a bit.
☐ No, I haven't exercised at all.
☐ I did some stuff, and that counts.

DETAILS

FOOD / MEDICATION

Food / Drinks	Meds / Supplements	Time	Dose

☐ usual daily medication

Notes

_____

I am grateful for...

M T W T F S S   DATE:

HOW ARE YOU *Feeling today?*

Amazing!	Meh
Great	Not good
Good	Terrible!

RATE YOUR PAIN LEVEL

① ② ③ ④ ⑤ ⑥ ⑦ ⑧ ⑨ ⑩

WHAT ABOUT YOUR...?

Mood	① ② ③ ④ ⑤ ⑥ ⑦ ⑧ ⑨ ⑩
Energy Levels	① ② ③ ④ ⑤ ⑥ ⑦ ⑧ ⑨ ⑩
Mental Clarity	① ② ③ ④ ⑤ ⑥ ⑦ ⑧ ⑨ ⑩

PAIN & SYMPTOM DETAILS

	am	pm	front	back	other
_____	☐	☐			☐ Nausea
_____	☐	☐			☐ Diarrhea
_____	☐	☐			☐ Vomiting
_____	☐	☐			☐ Sore throat
_____	☐	☐			☐ Congestion
_____	☐	☐			☐ Coughing
_____	☐	☐			☐ Chills
_____	☐	☐			☐ Fever

SLEEP

hours
_____

quality
① ② ③ ④ ⑤

STRESS LEVELS

None	Low	Medium	High	Max	@$#%!

WEATHER

☐ Cold ☐ Mild ☐ Hot
☐ Dry ☐ Humid ☐ Wet

Allergen Levels: _____
BM Pressure: _____

EXERCISE

☐ Heck yes, I worked out.
☐ I managed to exercise a bit.
☐ No, I haven't exercised at all.
☐ I did some stuff, and that counts.

DETAILS

FOOD / MEDICATION

Food / Drinks

Meds / Supplements	Time	Dose

☐ usual daily medication

Notes

_____

I am grateful for...

HOW ARE YOU *Feeling today?*

😍 Amazing!	🙂 Meh
😁 Great	😠 Not good
😊 Good	😵 Terrible!

RATE YOUR PAIN LEVEL

① ② ③ ④ ⑤ ⑥ ⑦ ⑧ ⑨ ⑩

WHAT ABOUT YOUR...?

Mood	① ② ③ ④ ⑤ ⑥ ⑦ ⑧ ⑨ ⑩
Energy Levels	① ② ③ ④ ⑤ ⑥ ⑦ ⑧ ⑨ ⑩
Mental Clarity	① ② ③ ④ ⑤ ⑥ ⑦ ⑧ ⑨ ⑩

PAIN & SYMPTOM DETAILS

	am	pm
_____	☐	☐
_____	☐	☐
_____	☐	☐
_____	☐	☐
_____	☐	☐
_____	☐	☐
_____	☐	☐
_____	☐	☐

front   *back*

other

- ☐ Nausea
- ☐ Diarrhea
- ☐ Vomiting
- ☐ Sore throat
- ☐ Congestion
- ☐ Coughing
- ☐ Chills
- ☐ Fever

SLEEP

hours
_____

quality
① ② ③ ④ ⑤

STRESS LEVELS

None	Low	Medium	High	Max	@$#%!

WEATHER

- ☐ Cold
- ☐ Dry
- ☐ Mild
- ☐ Humid
- ☐ Hot
- ☐ Wet

Allergen Levels: _____

BM Pressure: _____

EXERCISE

- ☐ Heck yes, I worked out.
- ☐ I managed to exercise a bit.
- ☐ No, I haven't exercised at all.
- ☐ I did some stuff, and that counts.

DETAILS

FOOD / MEDICATION

Food / Drinks

Meds / Supplements	Time	Dose

☐ usual daily medication

Notes
_____

_____

I am grateful for…

HOW ARE YOU *Feeling today?*

Amazing!	Meh
Great	Not good
Good	Terrible!

RATE YOUR PAIN LEVEL

① ② ③ ④ ⑤ ⑥ ⑦ ⑧ ⑨ ⑩

WHAT ABOUT YOUR...?

Mood	① ② ③ ④ ⑤ ⑥ ⑦ ⑧ ⑨ ⑩
Energy Levels	① ② ③ ④ ⑤ ⑥ ⑦ ⑧ ⑨ ⑩
Mental Clarity	① ② ③ ④ ⑤ ⑥ ⑦ ⑧ ⑨ ⑩

PAIN & SYMPTOM DETAILS

	am	pm	*front*	*back*	*other*
	☐	☐			☐ Nausea
	☐	☐			☐ Diarrhea
	☐	☐			☐ Vomiting
	☐	☐			☐ Sore throat
	☐	☐			☐ Congestion
	☐	☐			☐ Coughing
	☐	☐			☐ Chills
	☐	☐			☐ Fever

SLEEP

hours   *quality*
_____   ① ② ③ ④ ⑤

STRESS LEVELS

| None | Low | Medium | High | Max | @$#%! |

WEATHER

☐ Cold   ☐ Mild   ☐ Hot
☐ Dry   ☐ Humid   ☐ Wet
Allergen Levels: _____
BM Pressure: _____

EXERCISE

☐ Heck yes, I worked out.
☐ I managed to exercise a bit.
☐ No, I haven't exercised at all.
☐ I did some stuff, and that counts.

DETAILS

FOOD / MEDICATION

Food / Drinks

Meds / Supplements	Time	Dose

☐ usual daily medication

Notes
_____
_____

I am grateful for...

HOW ARE YOU *Feeling today?*

😍 Amazing!	🙂 Meh
😁 Great	😖 Not good
🙂 Good	😣 Terrible!

RATE YOUR PAIN LEVEL

①②③④⑤⑥⑦⑧⑨⑩

WHAT ABOUT YOUR...?

Mood	①②③④⑤⑥⑦⑧⑨⑩
Energy Levels	①②③④⑤⑥⑦⑧⑨⑩
Mental Clarity	①②③④⑤⑥⑦⑧⑨⑩

PAIN & SYMPTOM DETAILS

	am	pm	*front*	*back*	*other*
_____	☐	☐			☐ Nausea
_____	☐	☐			☐ Diarrhea
_____	☐	☐			☐ Vomiting
_____	☐	☐			☐ Sore throat
_____	☐	☐			☐ Congestion
_____	☐	☐			☐ Coughing
_____	☐	☐			☐ Chills
_____	☐	☐			☐ Fever

SLEEP

hours _____   *quality* ① ② ③ ④ ⑤

STRESS LEVELS

None	Low	Medium	High	Max	@$#%!

WEATHER

☐ Cold   ☐ Mild   ☐ Hot
☐ Dry   ☐ Humid   ☐ Wet
Allergen Levels: _____
BM Pressure: _____

EXERCISE

☐ Heck yes, I worked out.
☐ I managed to exercise a bit.
☐ No, I haven't exercised at all.
☐ I did some stuff, and that counts.

DETAILS

FOOD / MEDICATION

Food / Drinks

Meds / Supplements	Time	Dose

☐ usual daily medication

Notes
_____
_____

I am grateful for...

M T W T F S S DATE:

HOW ARE YOU *Feeling today?*

Amazing!	Meh
Great	Not good
Good	Terrible!

RATE YOUR PAIN LEVEL

① ② ③ ④ ⑤ ⑥ ⑦ ⑧ ⑨ ⑩

WHAT ABOUT YOUR...?

Mood	① ② ③ ④ ⑤ ⑥ ⑦ ⑧ ⑨ ⑩
Energy Levels	① ② ③ ④ ⑤ ⑥ ⑦ ⑧ ⑨ ⑩
Mental Clarity	① ② ③ ④ ⑤ ⑥ ⑦ ⑧ ⑨ ⑩

PAIN & SYMPTOM DETAILS

	am	pm	front	back	other
_____	☐	☐			☐ Nausea
_____	☐	☐			☐ Diarrhea
_____	☐	☐			☐ Vomiting
_____	☐	☐			☐ Sore throat
_____	☐	☐			☐ Congestion
_____	☐	☐			☐ Coughing
_____	☐	☐			☐ Chills
_____	☐	☐			☐ Fever

SLEEP

hours _____ *quality* ① ② ③ ④ ⑤

STRESS LEVELS

None	Low	Medium	High	Max	@$#%!

WEATHER

☐ Cold ☐ Mild ☐ Hot
☐ Dry ☐ Humid ☐ Wet

Allergen Levels: _____
BM Pressure: _____

EXERCISE

☐ Heck yes, I worked out.
☐ I managed to exercise a bit.
☐ No, I haven't exercised at all.
☐ I did some stuff, and that counts.

DETAILS

FOOD / MEDICATION

Food / Drinks

Meds / Supplements	Time	Dose

☐ usual daily medication

Notes

I am grateful for...

Notes

Made in the USA
Middletown, DE
20 December 2022

19992095R00106